P9-CRK-555

Yoga has helped **Fiona Agombar** in her recovery from ME – the most severe form of fatigue. She is a trustee of the charity Action for ME, and has been Assistant Editor of its magazine, *Interaction*.

Beat Fatigue with
<u>YOGA</u>

A STEP-BY-STEP GUIDE

Fiona Agombar

Element
An Imprint of HarperCollins*Publishers*
77–85 Fulham Palace Road
Hammersmith, London W6 8JB

The website address is: www.thorsons.com

First published in Great Britain in 1999 by
Element Books

1 3 5 7 9 10 8 6 4 2

© Fiona Agombar 1999

Fiona Agombar asserts the moral right to
be identified as the author of this work

Illustrations by David Woodroffe

A catalogue record for this book
is available from the British Library

ISBN 1 86204 352 6

Printed and bound in Great Britain by
Martins the Printers Limited, Berwick Upon Tweed

Contents

Illustrations

Acknowledgements

So many people have helped me with this project that I cannot possibly take all of the credit.

Firstly I would like to thank everybody at the Yoga for Health Foundation for their support and constructive advice, especially Howard Kent, Renée East and Eileen Nash. I would also like to thank my editor Grace Cheetham for having faith in this book, and for all her support. Also thanks to Ann Bryant, Gill Jacobs, Jayne Roscoe, Sally Graham and Dr Jonathan Briffa, who read my manuscript and made valuable comments. A special thank you is due to my husband Roy and my friend Annie Watsham who so painstakingly read through the first drafts and helped with the initial editing. The person I want to thank most, however, is Angela Stevens. Not only did Angela lead me to yoga, but she spent many hours reading my manuscript and giving her expert advice. This book would not be the same without her.

Foreword

Fiona Agombar has written a book which can – and I trust, will – do an immense amount of good. This is because she tells the story of her own experience and how, as she realized she was truly on a path to recovery, she then studied the background to and implications of this path.

The result is that we all can identify with this 20th-century business woman who fell into the traps set by our society, but who then was helped to the realization that she herself held the key to recovery. Her survey of the immense therapeutic power of yoga commands conviction because it comes not from a professional New Ager but from someone who was helped to see a vision and, by application, has turned that vision into a reality.

A Nobel prizewinner recently told a major medical conference that mankind's resistance to disease has declined markedly over the past half century. It is clear this decline is linked directly with the current 'Let-me-do-it-for-you' syndrome (which is also the 'Let-me-sell-it-to-you' syndrome). The immensely sophisticated and comprehensive human immune system developed naturally as central to man's self-help development, but today we are brainwashed to believe we must rely on others, or upon products, or upon technology, to keep us healthy. All these things have a role to play, but self-realization is at the core of our lives and we ignore this at our peril.

Having read Fiona's manuscript with real pleasure, it is certain that she is an excellent 'role model'. I keep this foreword brief because I do not want to delay you from reading a most rewarding text.

Howard Kent

Introduction

You're tired all the time, you're exhausted even – and you want to know how you can get more energy. Can this book help you? Well, I have witnessed many, many people with fatigue improve their quality of life dramatically by using yoga. With practice, you will become calmer, less stressed, and more content. In fact, if you really apply what you learn from this book, you will soon notice a huge improvement in your health and stamina.

Think about this. Wouldn't it be wonderful if you could tap into an endless source of energy? Wouldn't it be wonderful if you had so much vitality that you felt as if you were plugged into a main electricity circuit, rather than having a battery that runs flat all the time? *Yoga can help you tap into this energy – the universal energy that is all around us.* Quantum physics acknowledges that the universe consists of patterns of energy – of which atoms are a part. What you may not know is that the philosophy of yoga is based on the concept of how to use this energy, which is called *prana*, a Sanskrit word meaning the first unit of life force, or the energy which sustains all life and creation. Prana is said to be the sum total of all the energy that is manifest in the universe. Some say prana is to yoga what electricity is to modern civilization. Vigour, power, vitality, life and spirit are all forms of prana. This sounds almost too good to be true – can there really be such an energy force that we can discover? In this book we are going to look at prana, and I will show you how you can use this energy and gain endless vitality. There are some simple postures to practise, together with visualizations and breathing exercises that will dramatically increase your stamina – and really help *you* to beat fatigue. Like a car battery, you need to put yourself on charge to make use of this vital life force. If you can do this, you will have the key to mental and physical health. That is what this book is about – helping you to gain more energy and vitality through the use of special yoga exercises.

1

What Causes Fatigue?

One of the main reasons that you've bought this book may be because you feel tired for much of the time. But do you know *why* you feel tired – and how would you define how you feel? Is it that you generally feel 'below par', as if you are unable to function properly? Have you noticed a gradual drop in your energy levels? Do you feel unwell most of the time? Is this your only symptom? Or is your fatigue so severe that it interferes with your everyday life and actually stops you from working, or doing things that you usually enjoy? Whatever your symptoms, we will now look at the most common reasons for fatigue. Everybody feels tired if they over-exert themselves – this is normal. But stress, lifestyle, poor diet, doing too much and repeated infections on top of a run-down system can cause you to feel an unnatural tiredness. These factors can also lead to blocked *chakras*. In yoga, chakras are thought of as energy centres through which prana or universal energy is picked up. If they are not functioning properly you will feel very unwell. I'll explain more about prana and how you can work on your chakras to increase your energy levels in Chapter 3.

Please bear in mind that it's important to discuss your health with your doctor. Fatigue can be a sign that there is something seriously wrong. Cancer, heart disease, HIV, lupus, multiple sclerosis, rheumatoid arthritis, diabetes, an underactive thyroid and lung disease are just a few examples of what can cause serious exhaustion. However, fatigue that seems to have no cause is incredibly common. Dr Alan Stewart, in his book *Tired all the Time*, says that in the US fatigue accounts for 24 per cent of adults seeing their doctor. In fact, a report commissioned in the UK by the Royal Colleges of Physicians, Psychiatrists and General Practitioners in 1996 said: 'Fatigue is one of the most common complaints encountered in community health services.'

Fatigue often arises from the long-term running down of the body's system, so I'm going to start off by looking at stress. This is a very common cause of exhaustion – more common, in fact, than most of us realize.

LIFESTYLE AND STRESS

Stress can have a profound effect on your health at all levels and is one of the major reasons for fatigue. Strangely enough, you may not even be aware that you are under stress! So you do need to think about this. First of all, ask yourself: am I doing too much in my life? Am I actually taking out more than I am putting back in – in terms of making my own space in my life, having adequate rest and relaxation and proper nutrition? The way in which our bodies deal with pressure and strain – which is called our 'fight or flight' response – is not really equipped to cope with the stresses of modern-day living.

You may well have heard of the 'fight or flight' response. I'll explain it briefly, so that you can understand why, if it is constantly triggered, it can cause extreme tiredness. The first thing to understand is that it is what you think – your perception of an event – which triggers this response. Think about something that makes you very anxious now. You may feel your heart start to pound, your mouth go dry and your hands becoming clammy. You may notice butterflies in your tummy. This is because your digestive juices have slowed right down – which can create problems with absorbing the nutrients from your food – and this is one of the reasons why it is advisable to eat while you are calm and not under stress. So, how you think about an event affects your stress levels.

Our ancestors needed to have the 'fight or flight' response in order to deal with physical threats or emergencies – by running away from wild animals, for example. When your body is under stress, the autonomic part of your nervous system cuts in and your body leaps into action. This is largely unconscious – in other words, you have little control over what happens next. The hypothalamus gland in the brain, which monitors your systems, sends electrical and chemical messages to another part of your brain, the pituitary gland, which is largely responsible for hormone production in your body. A hormone called ACTH is then sent to the adrenal glands, which releases over 30 chemicals, including cortisol and adrenaline. (You know what this feels like – the speedy, anxious feeling you get from adrenaline!) In addition to all this, blood sugar is released from your liver into the blood in order to give a boost of energy; your blood pressure and heart rate rise; your digestive juices slow down or even stop (hence the dry mouth); the muscles of your neck and shoulders tense; you breathe faster and less deeply to take in more oxygen; and you perspire. This is all very well if you take the appropriate action – like running very fast – but it is not so good in a situation when you don't need this response. For example, if you are arguing with your boss or bank manager, or in a traffic jam, you don't need your blood pressure to rise or your breathing rate to change. The problem gets even worse if your body adapts to this 'fight or flight' response and doesn't relax afterwards – which it won't if you are constantly exposed to what *you* perceive as stressful situations. Later on I will show you how to control this potentially exhausting situation.

The Three Stages of Stress

The Canadian researcher Hans Selye noticed that the body goes through three stages when it is exposed to stress for a long time.

1 The Alarm Stage

This is the basic 'fight or flight' response as just described. When the body returns to normal you may feel very tired.

2 The Adaptation Stage

This is the stage I should like to concentrate on, and the stage at which you should start to take notice, before you pass into the third, more serious, stage. As you start to get used to being stressed, you may feel below par most of the time, because the 'fight or flight' mechanism is constantly switched on. The problem is, if you are under constant pressure, the nervous system is unable to bring the body back to its normal level. The worrying thing is that *you may not know that you are stressed and have reached this second stage, because you get used to living life at this pace.* This is why it is so important in yoga to learn to listen in to your body, so that you can take the appropriate action.

Some of the clues that you may have reached the Adaptation Stage include a sense of speeding up: talking and eating quite quickly, drinking fast and working at high speed. It's a bit like having your foot always on the accelerator pedal. This Adaptation Stage of stress is very tiring, as you are continually depleting your body of its natural reserves for the 'fight or flight' response. As you can imagine, you are likely to start to suffer from problems such as digestive disorders, high blood pressure, hyperventilation, anxiety, irritability and depression. You may have additional fatigue caused by low blood sugar as your adrenal glands start to become inefficient and the adrenaline can't keep your blood sugar level high enough. (Remember, the body is taking glucose from the liver.) Other problems that you may notice are that you become more susceptible to illness; you may suffer from mood swings, headaches, heart problems and insomnia. At this point, you will probably start relying on stimulants – like coffee, alcohol, cigarettes and sugary foods, even drugs – to get more energy. This is the worst thing you can do: your body needs better nutrition to support the adrenal glands, not stimulants to put a further burden on them!

3 The Exhaustion Stage

This is the final stage of continual stress, when the body has pushed itself too far and reaches the stage of utter exhaustion or burn-out. This is very serious as it can lead to total collapse, nervous breakdown, heart attack, ulcers, severe depression and anxiety, and severe fatigue. Doctors know the problems stress can create, but many of us are not willing to take the steps to do something about it. It is so much easier not to change our lifestyle and just to carry on, ignoring our symptoms.

Ways to Deal with Stress

- The first thing to do is to listen to your body and recognize if you are under stress. Once you start to see the familiar signs – such as tense muscles, fast respiration and a racing heartbeat – you can consciously practise relaxing your body and slowing down your breathing. This will bring down your heart rate and bring other symptoms of stress under control. (*See* the breathing exercises in Chapter 4.)
- Practise the Pose of Complete Rest (which you will find on page 33) every day. Try not to think of this as another thing that you need to make time for – think about it as your treat.
- Regular practice of yoga poses (which you will find in Chapters 5–8) will really help your stress levels.
- Whenever you feel under pressure, make a conscious effort to slow down your breathing and to breathe from your diaphragm (*see* page 17). Also, be aware of your posture.
- Meditate every day (*see* Chapter 9).
- Yoga helps bring balance into your life. The word yoga, meaning 'union', refers to the balance between mind, body and spirit – which I'll explain in more detail in Chapter 2. But you can think about balance in your life in terms of how much energy you use up and how much you put back in. Imagine that your stamina is like a bank account. You can't keep taking endlessly from your account – when you use up your energy, you must put something back into the account, like resting

between your daily activities, practising relaxation at least once a day, and eating nutritious food. You need to look after yourself!

- Eat a good diet. This is so important that I will refer to it constantly throughout this chapter. I will then explain what a good yoga diet is in more detail in the next chapter. Do remember for now that the more you suffer from stress, the more tempting it is to take short-cuts and to eat ready-prepared meals and junk food. Certain nutrients are required for the 'fight or flight' response, and if you are nutritionally deficient – or under constant stress – you may exhaust your adrenal system even more. Avoid sugar, alcohol, caffeine and stimulants.
- Start to be aware of how you think. Changing how you think will take a lot of practice. If you perceive a situation as negative, or with fear and anger, try to see the positive side of things. Of course this is easily said, but much more difficult to do. Is the situation teaching you a valuable lesson? Do you perhaps feel trapped, or feel that your life is hopeless and that you are stuck with something you hate – a job, relationship, financial commitment, or whatever? This is seldom true; change is always possible if you have the courage to recognize that you need to take action. Look at your lifestyle and how it is affecting your health. Resolve to make the changes that will reduce your stress levels if you can. Meanwhile, if you feel under pressure, thinking calm, healing thoughts is a powerful tool for coping with problems. Whenever something dreadful happens in my life I remind myself that I have to accept that some things can't be changed and that even pain eventually passes. We all have to learn to let go of the past and move on. Acceptance is not the same as putting up with a situation, but if you are calm, it is easier to see what action you could take to improve it. If you learn to control your emotions you will be in command of your feelings – not controlled by them. This is not the same as not showing your feelings – if you keep such a tight rein on them that you hide them, this will only increase your stress. Rather, allow your feelings to happen.

Accept what can't be changed, but control what can – as demonstrated by the third canoeist in the following analogy:

There were three canoeists on a rough sea. The first canoeist tried to steer against the sea with all his might. After a few hours he was completely exhausted and gave up; the sea overwhelmed him and he was drowned. The second canoeist didn't bother to fight the sea – he just let his canoe drift wherever the waves wanted to take him. He ended up being dashed onto the rocks. The third canoeist also knew he couldn't fight the sea – but he knew too that it would be foolish and weak just to drift. He used his paddle to steer a course, avoiding the rocks but harnessing the power of the sea to take him in the right direction, towards the safety of the harbour.

In this story, you are the canoeist and the sea is your life. You shouldn't fight and struggle against the things you can't change, but you do need to steer yourself in a positive direction if you want to avoid being overwhelmed with stress and tension.

A simple visualization
Lie down and close your eyes. Think very hard about anything that is making you feel unhappy or stressed. Now try to relax your body as much as you can. Imagine that you are blowing into a large red balloon. You are going to breathe all your stress into this balloon. Each time you breathe out, the balloon gets bigger. It is filling up with all your negative feelings. Anger, fear, hopelessness, grief, despair are all blown into the balloon. As the balloon gets larger, imagine you are tying it at the neck. Now let it go so it can start to float away. On each out-breath it goes further up into the sky, until you can't see it any more. Now, on each in-breath, breathe peace and calm into your body until it fills your whole being with relaxation.

Colin's Story

I am 60 and I work as a commercial manager dealing with legal and contract problems in the construction industry. I have always set myself very high standards of achievement – I am a real perfectionist. My philosophy has always been 'I must try my hardest', which I thought gave me a grip on life and my behaviour. In the last few years work had been getting more and more hectic. I guess I was suffering from all kinds of problems – a heart murmur, digestive problems, anxiety and fatigue – but I ignored these symptoms as much as I could. One day, on a particularly long journey, the traffic was atrocious and I decided I would stop at a friend's house. This I did, but suddenly my body seemed to take over and I felt completely drained of energy. I slept for four days without a break, and I still found I had no energy. I tried to go back to work, telling myself it was all in my mind, but I found it impossible to concentrate and I was completely physically drained. I couldn't seem to walk more than 30 or 40 yards.

By a series of coincidences, someone recommended that I attend a yoga retreat for a week. I was sceptical at first, but I went along to see what would happen. Practising yoga, meditation and relaxation slowly built up my energy. My body felt in tune with the yoga postures and every day a light shone brighter. I went home and took another three weeks rest before I returned to work. During this time I realized the importance of discipline, and I practised yoga every morning for 40 minutes. Each day I had a period of meditation and relaxation. This all energized me. Now, every day I practise yoga and meditate and seem to be in complete control of my life. At work, I take a break at lunchtime and have a walk. I try to follow a diet based on the yoga principles. I feel ten years younger, happy, and at peace with all that surrounds me. My world is full of love for all people and the universe. You may think it sounds like a cliché – but when I found yoga it was a turning point in my life!

OTHER CONDITIONS AFFECTING ENERGY LEVELS

Allergies and Intolerances

Usually, if you are allergic to a food or substance, your immune system will respond in such a way that you will have a severe reaction. A true allergy invokes the response of your immune system, usually raising histamine levels. This means that after eating the offending food, or breathing in a chemical or pollen that you are allergic to, you may have a violent reaction – such as a skin rash, streaming eyes or a runny nose. Examples of this kind of allergy include eczema, asthma and coeliac disease (an allergy to gluten). However, it is becoming increasingly common for people to develop food or environmental sensitivities. As a result of a low-grade chronic immune response, you may experience symptoms you find difficult to define – mood disorders, concentration difficulties, breathing problems, weight fluctuations, erratic heartbeat, skin disorders, joint problems, irritable bowel syndrome – and fatigue.

Allergies and food or chemical intolerances are more common today because our immune systems have to put up with so much more than they did 50 years ago. Pesticides, food additives, antibiotics and pollution are just a few of the things that can challenge and overload your immune system. By this I mean that the defence system of your body is so overworked that it can't cope as effectively and eventually breaks down. A poor diet can add to this picture – if you are not eating properly you are not supporting your immune system and helping it to cope. Stress can also increase the likelihood of your developing allergies or food sensitivities – if you are eating when stressed, your body is not producing enough digestive juices to help with the proper absorption of food. Worse, if you develop candida, which I shall discuss later on, you may suffer from leaky-gut syndrome which means that undigested particles of foods can pass through your gut wall. This may cause your immune system to over-react, because it sees these food particles as foreign bodies – or allergens. Yet again, you can see that diet has a vital contribution to make in beating fatigue.

If you can identify the substances to which you are sensitive and avoid them, this can greatly help your energy levels. However, this can be difficult because if you continue to eat a substance to which you are intolerant, your body will adapt and the reactions become less severe and more vague. It then becomes difficult to identify the offending food – it is easier to detect when you have a more obvious and severe allergic response. Worse still, you may even crave the foods that your body is sensitive to! This is because you will get a temporary lift as adrenaline is produced to fight the reaction. However, this beneficial effect disappears after a couple of hours and you may then feel unwell again.

The best way to discover if you suffer from food or chemical sensitivities is to go on a modified fast for five days. This gives your body time to rest. You will then be able to 'unmask' culprit foods when you reintroduce them gradually, because if you do have an intolerance, you will have a more severe reaction when you next eat the offending food. This is best done under supervision – but both *The Elimination Diet Cookbook* and *The Rotation Diet Cookbook* (which explains the benefits of varying and rotating your diet to avoid food intolerance) by Jill Carter and Alison Edwards, will tell you how to tackle allergies and intolerances. It will also help if you eat only organic food, use unperfumed products in the house and bathroom, and avoid pollution and sprays wherever possible; you are then not putting such a load on your immune system.

Anaemia

Anaemia refers to a deficiency in the blood (usually of red blood cells) or low levels of haemoglobin (the red blood pigment that contains iron and carries oxygen around the body). Anaemia is not caused just by an iron deficiency. It may be due to a lack of copper, folic acid, or vitamins B_{12} and C. It is usually a gradual process – as your red cell activity moves slowly away from its normal range – until you notice that you feel tired and run down. If you are anaemic, check with your doctor and supplement your diet with vitamins C, B$_{12}$, and folic acid as well as iron.

Candida

You may have heard about candida as it has received a lot of attention in recent years. If you are suffering from fatigue it certainly is something you should consider, because it could be causing your fatigue. *Candida albicans* is a yeast-like mould which lives in all of us. It lives on the skin and in mucous membranes such as the digestive tract. Usually there is no problem with this as it is kept in check by friendly bacteria. The problem arises only when there are not enough of these friendly bacteria. A number of factors contribute to candida overgrowth: antibiotics (which kill off the bacteria), the contraceptive pill (which affects hormone function; candida thrives when progesterone is high), steroid drugs, a weakened immune system, stress, and poor nutrition (such as a diet high in sugar). The situation is made worse if candida gets a grip on your digestive system and puts down root-like structures which can cause your gut to leak – allowing partly digested foods to pass into your bloodstream. This can then cause you to become sensitive to certain foods, which may well compound your tiredness (as explained in the section under allergies). As the candida dies off, it gives off toxins that can make you feel very unwell.

The symptoms of candida include severe fatigue, headaches, itchy anus, thrush, constipation and diarrhoea, food cravings, mood swings, difficulty in concentrating, foggy head, bloating and gas. It may also cause irritable bowel syndrome. You may have some of these symptoms – you are unlikely, or very unlucky, if you have them all. If you suspect you have candida, do see a practitioner who can test you and give you the appropriate treatment. This will involve following a diet which excludes all forms of sugar, yeast and alcohol, and supplements to help kill off the candida and repopulate the gut with friendly bacteria. After this regime, your energy levels should improve dramatically. *Beat Candida Through Diet* by Gill Jacobs and Joanna Kjaer, and *The Natural Way with Candida* by Simon Martin are good books to read if you want to find out more about treating Candida.

Chronic Fatigue Syndrome

Chronic Fatigue Syndrome (CFS) is an umbrella term to describe a collection of symptoms, including very serious fatigue. There has been much argument over the definition of CFS in recent years – for example, some doctors include psychiatric illnesses such as depression and somatoform disorders (a physical illness caused by a mental problem), whereas others do not. In yoga, mind, body and spirit all need to be in balance for good health – and each has a role in any illness. Having said this, research has shown that most people with CFS do *not* have a psychiatric condition. Of course, psychological factors can develop as a secondary problem in any long-term chronic illness. The most severe form of CFS is known as ME (Myalgic Encephalomyelitis) in the UK and CFIDS (Chronic Fatigue Immune Dysfunction Syndrome) in the US. CFS is also known as Post Viral Fatigue – that is, the profound fatigue you may suffer after having a viral illness such as flu.

If you suffer from fatigue, you have probably wondered at some time if you are suffering from Chronic Fatigue Ssyndrome. CFS is usually defined as a long-term fatigue that lasts for six or more months, with severe exhaustion following even minor physical or mental exertion. If you suffer from CFS you will certainly know about it – even moving a limb or doing a simple task such as having a bath or cooking a meal may seem like climbing a mountain. It is total physical and mental exhaustion – like a battery that has gone completely flat. Worse, you don't just feel tired (which is what most people think CFS is), you feel very unwell for much of the time. Symptoms may include a foggy head and difficulty in concentrating, sleep disturbance, muscle aches or spasms, a feeling of being poisoned, and sensitivity to light and noise. If your fatigue really is CFS, you will notice that these symptoms fluctuate. On some days you may feel well – you may even have good weeks. Usually you will feel better in the morning and worse as the day progresses. In any case, you will find it impossible to cope with your previous level of lifestyle – most people who have CFS have to give up work and severely curtail their social activities. The UK charity, Action for ME, describes CFS as being like trying to run a marathon with flu and a hangover. My own definition is that simple tasks can sometimes feel like trying to swim through treacle after having done ten rounds in a boxing ring!

Several factors may cause CFS. It may be triggered by a virus, by shock, by inoculation, by exposure to environmental toxins, or it may be the final stage of adrenal exhaustion due to continued stress. The cause may be only one of these factors, or several combined. Whatever causes it, CFS can have a devastating effect on your life, and it may take several years before you recover. For this reason, you need to be able to deal with your emotions, which at times you may find overwhelming. Many people who have CFS find that they experience a kind of grief – a sense of loss for their old way of life and who they were before they became ill. You should expect to experience shock, disbelief and, later on, anger. These are all normal emotions under the circumstances. If you have had CFS for several years, you will eventually be able to accept your changed circumstances. Often, it is at this point that you start to recover – when you are no longer fighting against the illness but are able to accept that this is how you are for now and that you have to make the best of what you have.

If you have CFS the big question is whether you can exercise or not. Sometimes people are advised to have complete rest, whereas others are put on a graded exercise programme, so the subject is very controversial. This is where yoga can play a vital role in your recovery, *because you can do yoga postures at your own rate – according to your level of health*. There is no competition in yoga, so you do not have to push yourself into a relapse. Yoga helps with the recovery process since it forms a very strong foundation for getting better. The first step is learning to listen to your body so that you can take note of how you feel and pace yourself properly. Work out your own yoga programme according to your level of health. You may start just with breathing, stretching and meditation. The key with CFS is never to overdo things – always do less than you think you can do. For example, if you feel well enough to do 20 minutes of yoga postures, do only 10 minutes; if you feel you can do only 10 minutes, then do five. Five minutes is better than no minutes and is a base on which to build. Aim to work slowly, to add perhaps an extra posture every month. Don't be tempted to do too much on a good day. If you are having a bad day, or a relapse, or are very ill, then practise just the relaxation and breathing exercises. The postures are of great benefit because as well as keeping your whole system going, they create extra oxygen in your blood so that your cells can burn up the food you have eaten and convert it into energy. In CFS you may experience the additional problem of muscle wastage because of long-term inactivity. This will make you feel even more exhausted if you try to do anything. As long as you build up your muscle tolerance slowly; set yourself small, achievable goals; pace yourself; keep to your limits and are patient; you will find that gentle yoga helps tremendously. The road back to good health will be long and slow – but yoga will take you in the right direction.

I would strongly advise you not to join an ordinary yoga class until you have made considerably progress in your recovery; it is too easy to over-do things and relapse. Either join a remedial class or follow the postures in this book that you feel well enough to do at home. (Details of how to find a suitable yoga class can be found in the Useful Addresses Section.) If you would like to know more about CFS, a good book to read is *The Natural Way: Chronic Fatigue Syndrome* by Gill Jacobs, details of which are given in the Bibliography.

Depression

I have already explained that you may not know you are suffering from stress, because you adapt to it. Likewise, you may not know that you are suffering from depression. This may sound like an amazing statement, but doctors know that sufferers of depression can fail to realize that their mood has gradually lowered, until they find their world utterly hopeless and grey. I mention depression here because it is a very common cause of fatigue – so common that many doctors still confuse it with Chronic Fatigue Syndrome. Unfortunately it is something most people are ashamed to admit – as if in some way it is their fault, which it isn't. Depression is often caused by how you view the world. Does your fantasy of how life should be match life as it really is? This is where yoga can help: yoga teaches us acceptance of how life is; it shows us the illusion of things such as materialism, and teaches us to live more in the present and not to catastrophize about what may – or may not – happen.

Depression may be caused by stress, so if you think you have a problem with low mood, look again at the suggestions given on coping with stress. Symptoms of depression may include weight gain or loss, insomnia, anxiety, loss of interest in life and other people, feelings of worthlessness, a sense of having failed in life and a sense of being bored and dissatisfied with life. Depression can lead to self-criticism to the extent of losing confidence and self-esteem. If you suspect you are depressed you must seek medical help. Lack of exercise can add to the problem, so try to set small goals for yourself and practise a few yoga postures every day. Nutrition can dramatically affect your mood – for example, lack of the B vitamins and amino acids found in protein can contribute towards depression, as can sugar, caffeine and alcohol. Following the diet recommended in Chapter 2 will help elevate your energy and mood.

Hormone Imbalance

We looked at some of the hormones that affect fatigue when we examined stress – adrenaline and insulin were just two that were mentioned. Your hormones can have a profound effect on your energy levels. If you are a woman and you suffer from premenstrual syndrome (PMS), you will know that this is true! Men are also affected by their hormones. Your hormone or endocrine system is largely controlled by the pituitary gland in your brain. There are various hormones, the imbalance of which can bring about changes in the body's chemistry, leading to symptoms including mood changes and fatigue. Your hormone balance can be affected by various lifestyle factors such as diet and exercise and getting out of rhythm with your cycles. For example, if you go to bed during the day and not at night, your pituitary gland will eventually stop producing the hormone melatonin at the right time to help you sleep – and this will have a knock-on effect on other hormones. I'll talk more about rhythm in the next chapter.

One hormone worth mentioning here is thyroxine, produced by the thyroid gland. If your thyroid gland is not producing enough thyroxine, your body will be unable to convert your food into energy. Thyroxine stimulates the body's cells to take in more oxygen to help with this conversion. The symptoms of hypothyroidism (an underactive thyroid) include weight gain, undue sensitivity to cold, aches and pain – and fatigue. Your thyroid function can be checked with a simple blood test. There is a current theory that people who suffer from Chronic Fatigue Syndrome (CFS) will often show a test result at the lower end of the normal range – and that they get better with a low dose of thyroxine. By all means check with your doctor if you think having a hormone test will help, but meanwhile practise your yoga postures and eat a balanced diet with sufficient protein.

Hyperventilation

I have already mentioned that you may not be aware that you are suffering from certain states, such as stress and depression. The same can be said for hyperventilation, which can also cause profound fatigue. It is very common, but if you are suffering from hyperventilation, it is very unlikely that you will be aware that this is a problem.

Hyperventilation is defined as breathing at a rate greater than your body needs. People who hyperventilate tend not to use their diaphragm when they breathe, but breathe only from their upper chest area. When we talk about breathing it is vital that you understand exactly what your diaphragm is and what it does. It is a large sheet of muscle attached to your spine at the back, and to your bottom ribs at the front. When you breathe in, your diaphragm ensures that your lungs are fully inflated (*see* figure 1). When you breathe out, your diaphragm rises in a cone

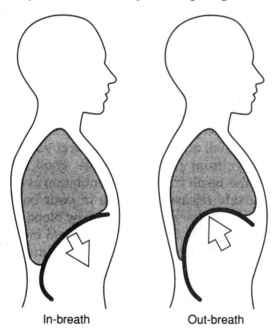

In-breath   Out-breath

Figure 1   Movement of the diaphragm

shape, so you can see that it acts like a piston. When your posture is good and your muscles properly in balance, your diaphragm can help to balance and relax your body. You'll see why this is later, when you read the section on posture.

Most people think that they need lots of oxygen for energy. What you actually need is a balance of oxygen and carbon dioxide, and if you breathe too fast you breathe off too much carbon dioxide. What then happens is that the pH of the blood gradually becomes too alkaline. This can have a serious effect on your muscles and nerves. Also, if you shallow breathe, your levels of magnesium will be used up, and magnesium deficiency has been shown to be a contributing factor in Chronic Fatigue Syndrome. Symptoms that may indicate that you are hyperventilating include talking too fast, vivid dreams, a tingling numbness in your hands, difficulty in getting your breath, yawning and sighing a lot, and difficulty in swallowing. As the problem becomes more severe you may eventually experience panic attacks, phobic states, and a feeling of being 'spaced out' or unreal.

Hyperventilation may be caused by stress – you will remember that when the 'fight or flight' mechanism kicks in, your breathing rate increases (*see* figure 2.) You will also remember that if you are under constant pressure, this mechanism may not shut down completely, so that you will continue to breathe fast and your body will get used to breathing in this way. Because breathing too rapidly activates adrenaline, you will also find that it makes you very tense, and you may suffer from painful muscles. Food intolerance and allergies can also result from hyperventilation as the lower levels of carbon dioxide release histamine in your body, which may contribute towards allergic reactions. Low blood sugar and poor posture can also add to the picture of a rapid breathing pattern.

Your breathing is largely driven by your unconscious, *but you can override it and learn to breathe properly*. If you are breathing more than 18 times a minute, you are probably breathing too fast. Try to slow down to a cycle of 12 breaths a minute. Practise this for 10 minutes, twice a day. Remember to breathe through your nose if you can – which will stop you breathing in great gulps of air. In

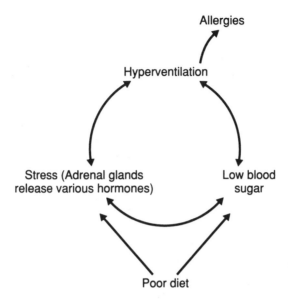

Figure 2   The hyperventilation cycle

yoga you should always breathe through your nose anyway, as the fine hairs in your nostrils help to filter out toxins. Although it may be necessary to breathe fast if you are being chased by a wild animal, it is inappropriate in most everyday situations, such as in a traffic jam or in an argument with someone!

Hypoglycaemia

Hypoglycaemia literally means a low level of sugar in the blood. It is a very common cause of fatigue – especially now that some nutritionists are encouraging people to eat lots of carbohydrates and saying that certain combinations of food – protein and starches, for example – should not be eaten together (food combining). However, if you don't eat enough protein and complex carbohydrates in combination, this can lead to the state of low blood sugar or hypoglycaemia. As with stress, it is very possible to suffer from this condition without realizing it.

We all need glucose for energy, and our body converts the food we eat into glucose so that it can be used for our brain and nervous system. On a reasonable diet, this conversion takes place over a period of several hours from the breakdown of fats, proteins and carbohydrates. Your blood sugar level lies within a certain normal range under these conditions. When you eat, this level rises as you absorb the glucose from your food – then it falls back to normal. The problem starts when your blood sugar level rises too high, too quickly – and this will happen if you eat sweet, sugary food or fast-releasing carbohydrates such as white pasta, cakes or white rice. These foods are converted to glucose much faster than proteins and complex starches, such as brown rice or products made with wholegrain flour. What then happens is that your pancreas tries to compensate for this steep rise in blood sugar by releasing insulin, which tries to push your glucose into the body's cells. In this way glycogen and insulin are competing to stabilize your blood sugar level. But if it has gone too high, the insulin will make it drop – sometimes very low, below the normal range.

The symptoms which you may experience to tell you if this is happening include irritability (especially before a meal), nausea, faintness, weakness, dizziness, lack of concentration, shakiness, headaches, anxiety, mood swings and an overwhelming desire to binge. You will also feel very tired. You are also likely to hyperventilate, which will add to the picture of stress and fatigue – hyperventilation and low blood sugar are connected. You may have only some of these symptoms. You are especially likely to feel like this between meals, mid to late morning and mid to late afternoon, for example. You will then crave and eat sugary foods to give you a quick lift. You may crave to the point of addiction – you *have* to have that chocolate bar, glass of wine or jam doughnut! A couple of hours later you will feel very tired as your blood sugar level drops again. Incidentally, this is why dieters often fail – if they don't eat properly and become hypoglycaemic, they have overwhelming desires to binge so as to raise their low blood sugar level. To add to this picture, if you have low blood sugar your body produces more adrenaline, which puts a strain on your adrenal system. This can trigger the 'fight or flight' response, giving you a false feeling of energy and alertness, which in the long run is very tiring. So, indirectly, being hypoglycaemic will add to any stress or tiredness you are experiencing – and vice versa (*see* figure 2).

The way to break the roller coaster pattern of high/low blood sugar is very simple. You need to aim to keep your blood sugar level stable. This will take only a few days, during which time you may crave sweet foods – but stick with it, as the results can be remarkable.

- Always eat some form of protein with your starches. So don't have a piece of toast or crisp bread on its own, but have something like cottage cheese, tahini or almond butter with it. Don't eat just a jacket potato and salad, but have them with a protein such as pulses or fish. The Hay diet, which recommends keeping protein and starches separate, may work for some people, but if you are hypoglycaemic, it is a bad idea.
- Eat every 3–4 hours. Good snacks include nuts and seeds.
- Avoid coffee and alcohol – they will make your problem worse.
- Avoid sweets and sugar at all costs. Do not eat food that contains white flour or white rice. Buns, cakes and desserts are out.
- Don't miss meals and always eat a good breakfast that includes some form of protein.
- Physical exercise improves blood sugar control, so practise your yoga postures.

Low blood pressure

People talk a lot about the problems of high blood pressure. However, if you have low blood pressure this will make you feel dizzy and fatigued. Low blood pressure is actually considered a medical condition in Germany, although in other countries it is considered normal, even though it can leave you feeling tired and weak. If your blood pressure is low, the inverted yoga postures (such as the Shoulder Stand) described in Chapter 8 will help.

HOW POSTURE AFFECTS ENERGY LEVELS

Correct posture is so important that I want to explain how it affects your health at all levels. You will then see how the yoga poses will give you more energy as your posture improves. When you are tired, you are more likely to flop or slump in your chair. Unfortunately, this will make you more tired as major organs of your body become restricted. Your heart will beat faster and your rib area will tense so that you can't breathe properly – and this will make your thoughts race. This then becomes a vicious circle – the more fatigued you become, the more you slump, until you are almost curling into yourself, which in turn can make you feel more exhausted and depressed!

The health of your spine is essential for your wellbeing. Not only does it support your body, but it also contains the spinal cord, the main route for information from the nervous system to the brain. The cerebrospinal fluid contained in the spinal cord provides the brain and nerve tissues with oxygen and nutrition, and helps with the drainage of waste products. Amazingly, this fluid has a physical potency of energy with its own rhythm and pulsation – which fluctuates at 10–14 cycles per minute in healthy adults. Fear can actually stop this fluid from flowing! The cerebrospinal fluid is also vulnerable to outside influences such as tea, coffee and stress – and, of course, poor posture.

The cerebrospinal fluid affects the biochemistry of every cell in the body and plays an important role in internal tissue respiration. Any disturbance in the spinal fluid may show in your breathing – and so yoga breathing can help in keeping this fluid healthy. An osteopath who uses the sacrocranial technique works with the pulsation of the spinal fluid and its link to the brain. When your cerebrospinal fluid is flowing properly, your energy levels will be enhanced.

Poor posture restricts the digestion. If your colon is compressed it is difficult for it to function efficiently and you may suffer from all kinds of digestive disorders, including Irritable Bowel Syndrome. If you slump, you also restrict your diaphragm, which can lead to all kinds of problems. If you can't breathe properly, you will probably start to hyperventilate, which in turn can affect your mental outlook and energy levels. (On a visit to a psychiatric hospital I noticed all the patients had terrible posture – some were slumped very far forward. I wonder if their posture contributed to their condition – or was it the other way around?) Without doubt, if you start to slump forward, you will feel more depressed and fatigued. Poor posture also leads to tense muscles, which also will drain your energy. Most of the time we are unaware of the tension we hold in our back. If you put your arm out and make a tight fist, and hold it for 10 seconds, you will start to understand how much energy tight muscles use up. What you want to aim for is a posture that involves no tension, so that you are relaxed at all times of the day.

Poor posture restricts the blood flow so that eventually there is less oxygen reaching your cells and the blood is unable to nourish them; also, it squashes your abdominal organs – all of which will make you feel exhausted. Think about how you are sitting now. Are you slumped so that the area around your navel is compressed? Is there any tension in your back? Check to see if the bottom end of your breast-bone is lifted away from your abdomen – just making this tiny correction will help. Aiming for better posture will definitely give you lots more energy.

The yoga postures or *asanas* will help to keep your spinal column and the cerebrospinal fluid healthy. The asanas also supply nutrients and fluids to your spinal discs. If they do not receive them, the discs become hard and start to degenerate. The spinal twists and backward bends described in later chapters will greatly help your back. As the yoga poses improve the strength of your spine, your breathing and digestion as well as your posture will improve. This in turn will improve your mental faculties – you will feel more energized and alert and your concentration will be better. For more information on perfect posture, *see* the Mountain Pose in Chapter 7.

SUMMARY

As you will see in the next chapter, yoga sees us as a whole – not just a collection of individual parts. So although I've talked about various parts – such as your digestive system, adrenal function, endocrine system and respiration system – yoga aims to work on your whole system in order to bring everything back into balance, so that you can experience good health. Remember too that you need to work on this harmony in your life – you need to balance work with relaxation and to have balance in your diet. My recipe for combating fatigue is as follows:

- Practise the yoga postures given later – every day if possible.
- Take enough rest and relaxation.
- Eat a very nutritious diet and drink plenty of water.
- Practise the yoga breathing techniques given in Chapter 4. Check your own breathing rate.
- Sit outside in the sunshine when you can – we take in prana or energy from the food we eat, the air we breathe and from sunshine.
- Meditate for 20 minutes a day – *see* Chapter 9.
- Try and develop a positive attitude; set yourself goals in life so that you know in which direction you are going.

I hope this has given you a better insight into what may be causing your fatigue – and some suggestions for how to tackle the problem. In the following chapters we will look more closely at yoga and see what it has to offer in terms of increasing your energy levels.

2

An Introduction to Yoga

The last chapter should have given you some idea about what is causing you to feel tired. In this chapter I will introduce you to yoga and explain how it can help you to have much more vitality. Put simply, yoga *will* help you to beat fatigue, however it is caused, because yoga is all about using prana. As I explained in the Introduction, prana is the first unit of life force, or the energy which sustains all life. Prana is said to be the total of *all* the energy in the universe.

Although our bodies are saturated with prana (it is absorbed from the air, the sun and the food we eat), our vitality depends on how we are able to use this energy. Yoga will help you to control, direct and store prana. As you will discover later, yoga postures and exercises will help you to balance your own energy centres, or chakras, so that your prana can flow properly. Your chakras take in this universal energy via the *nadis* (another Sanskrit word), which are channels like electric circuits. When your own energy is not flowing as it should, you become ill because prana cannot flow through the body. I'll be discussing prana and chakras in more detail in the next chapter, but for now you should understand that in yoga the traditional way for waking up this energy is through breath control, meditation and physical postures.

THE UNITY OF MIND, BODY AND SPIRIT

Yoga is also about the *balance* of your physical, mental and spiritual states, and about how to bring these states into harmony. In yoga, we look at the whole system without trying to break the body up into separate parts. Your state of mind, for example, will affect your immune and endocrine (hormone) system, which in turn will affect your circulation and breathing – and so on. In other words it is impossible to look at any one part of the body in isolation. If you really want to beat fatigue and gain perfect health, you need to look at not just your physical requirements – which so much of Western living seems to concentrate on – but at your mental and spiritual needs as well. In this way, yoga sees a unity between mind, body and spirit. But what do we understand by 'mind', 'body' and 'spirit'? The late 20th century places little importance on their interconnection. Most of us take too little exercise, suffer from an overload of stress and tension, and live in a society where the emphasis is on the material, not the spiritual.

Mind

According to Patanjali, an Indian sage who wrote about yoga around 2,000 years ago: 'Yoga is the control of thought waves of the mind.' This may surprise you if you thought that yoga was just a series of exercises. In fact, Patanjali was making a very powerful statement. After all, an unquiet mind is very exhausting – it would be wonderful if you could learn how to control it. In yoga, a restless mind is likened to a chattering monkey, or the ripples on an otherwise calm lake. If you are mentally tense you may suffer from racing thoughts, have a tendency to be over-emotional, or you may experience anxiety and phobias, or even depression. All of this will deplete your energy. Practising yoga will put you back in the driving seat and help you to be calm and in control.

A thought *is* energy, and so how you think is very important for your health. Because you *are* what you think, working on the mind has a profound effect on the body. In yoga this is achieved, as you will see in later chapters, through relaxation, concentration and visualization exercises, learning to breathe properly and, ultimately, by meditation.

An example of how your mind can control your energy levels is demonstrated by the following experiment, which I have witnessed several times. It was devised by Howard Kent, who runs the Yoga for Health Foundation in the UK and who is well known for having popularized yoga in the West in the early 1970s. He asks two volunteers to hold their arms out vertically. He then pushes on their arms to see how much resistance there is. One volunteer is then asked to think of 'nothing in particular', while the other is told to think of the mantra 'I breathe in life and energy' for one minute. Howard then pushes on the arms again. The arm of the person who has been thinking of nothing gives way easily, but the person who has been repeating the mantra finds he has the muscle strength to resist the pressure on his arm. So thinking positively *can* directly affect your muscle strength.

In another experiment – conducted when it was snowing outside – the central heating was turned off in Howard's office and the temperature fell to about 2°C. Howard was then wrapped in wet towels. His aim was to dry the towels with the heat of his body – which he did in about two and three-quarter hours. Most people would have suffered from hypothermia! When I asked him how and why he had done this, he said: 'I wanted to *prove* that the mind can control the body. All I did was to imagine I was in Tuscany, lying in the hot sun. This shows that a mental image can be stronger than a physical "fact". It also shows how you can use the power of the mind to create your own reality.'

Body

Yoga postures help tremendously on a physical level because they both conserve and give energy – unlike ordinary exercise, such as jogging or aerobics, which actually uses up energy. Yoga helps your body because it:

- tones the muscles
- delays ageing
- benefits the joints and skeleton
- strengthens the circulation, heart and lung capacity – oxygenates the blood better and improves breathing
- improves digestion
- strengthens the back and makes the spine more flexible – so helps posture
- balances the nervous system – so helps to relax the whole body
- balances the endocrine system – so helps with hormone levels
- nourishes all organs and glands
- balances the chakras (your energy centres)
- cleanses and removes toxins
- gives energy

Spirit

Spiritual balance is fundamental to yoga practice. Spirit can perhaps best be defined as being anything that is *not* physical – such as the abstract part of your being that you can nourish through love. For example, and to put this more simply, if you have a love of nature and of music or art, then you probably have an idea of what is spiritual. Living in the moment, or doing creative things like painting or listening to music, can help you to find this, because when you get lost in such tasks you are experiencing a universal unity. By this I mean that you forget yourself and who you are as you become absorbed in the creative process. We will examine this in more detail when we look at meditation in Chapter 9.

A lack of spiritual direction can lead to depression, fear, anxiety and a loss of purpose in life. Listening in with yoga helps you to connect with your soul, spirit, or inner self. It is about coming into balance with the Universal Life Force, or whatever you feel comfortable calling it. This will give you tremendous energy, for being spiritually depleted is very draining.

LISTEN IN TO THE RHYTHM OF YOUR BODY

Rhythm is fundamental to our wellbeing. Your body has its own rhythm: you have your own breathing rhythm, your own monthly cycle (men as well as women), and your own heartbeat rhythm. If you think about it, the earth also has its own rhythm. There is the cycle of the seasons, the cycle of the moon and the cycle of day following night. This last cycle affects us profoundly. Our master gland, the hypothalamus – which is in the brain and controls many of our functions – actually secretes hormones depending on whether it is light or· dark. Chronobiology, the science of looking at biological rhythms, accepts that our bodies have an in-built rhythm of their own. As Dr Andrew Wright, medical advisor for the charity Action for ME, says: 'Health is dependent on the rhythmical changes of these in-built cycles imposing order on the body, thereby enforcing stability through change! Rhythms are so much a part of our lives, be they in music or dance or whatever, that it is not surprising that they play a part in keeping us well.'

Yoga is about self-awareness, and our awareness of natural rhythms is so often lost or numbed by the stresses in our current way of living. Our ancestors lived in harmony with the planet – they got up when the sun rose, went to bed at sunset, and ate local foods that were in season. Modern-day living has made us lose touch with these rhythms, so before you begin your yoga postures, it is important to develop this awareness.

Developing Awareness Exercise
This is a very simple exercise which involves no physical exertion. First of all, ask yourself how you *feel* right now as you

are reading this. Are you tired, interested, bored or energized? Do you feel well today? Now listen to the way you breathe and try to slow it down. Are you breathing only from the upper chest area? Is your heart beating fast or slow? Stop and think about this for a while.

Then start to think about the way you move. For example, when you are walking up stairs, try breathing in as you slowly lift your leg up, and out as you put it down. In this way you are starting to introduce rhythm into your movements – an awareness of *how* you move. You can also practise moving in time with you breath whenever you are out walking. Try breathing in as your walk for four steps, then out as you walk for four more steps.

Finally, consider what you eat. Do you buy local produce that is in season and – if possible – organic? Start to become more aware of yourself – how you actually *feel* (well, unwell, tired, happy, sad) – and start thinking about how you treat your body. Do you take your health for granted, eat lots of junk food and take little exercise, for example? As you start to notice yourself more by paying attention to your body and your health, you will start to develop inner awareness.

THE EIGHT LIMBS OF YOGA

Yoga is very much about taking control and responsibility for your own health. As Patanjali explained, yoga is about controlling the mind. Patanjali saw illness as a state of imbalance that creates a negative energy which in turn dims our prana; our life force. He said that such things as disease, sluggishness, carelessness, living in the world of illusion (ie not accepting things as they really are), sorrow, despair, anger, being miserable, and poor breathing will create this imbalance. Of course, this is a never-ending cycle – if you are miserable and angry you won't have the energy to think positively! So Patanjali devised The Eight Limbs of Yoga to help break this cycle and achieve perfect health, ready for enlightenment. The eight limbs are as follows (with their Sanskrit names or English equivalent):

1 A code of universal ethics to be followed, known as the *yama*
2 A code of personal conduct, called *niyama*
3 The practice of physical postures, known as *asana*
4 The practice and control of prana through yoga breathing – *pranayama*
5 The practice of learning to control and withdraw the senses
6 Concentration – learning to still the mind
7 Meditation
8 Enlightenment

Some people think of the Eight Limbs of Yoga as a ladder – or something that you learn in order of progression. This is not really true; all the limbs are important and form part of the whole concept of yoga. However, most people start yoga at step three and learn the postures that exercise the body and relax the mind. After regular practice of this, and perhaps step four – breath control – you will realize other changes are happening. Your attitude to life will start to shift as you become more balanced and in harmony with your true self. This may then lead you on to examine steps one and two – the yamas and niyamas. You may find that you start to become more thoughtful and compassionate and less ruled by your desires, and so you move on to step five – the withdrawal of your senses. As your concentration becomes better and your mind calmer, you are ready for meditation.

In this book, because we are dealing specifically with fatigue, we will be concentrating on the third limb (the yoga postures), the fourth limb (yoga breathing) and the seventh limb (meditation).

Asanas – the yoga postures

The third limb of yoga comprises the yoga postures, or asanas. This is how most people think of yoga – as a form of exercise – but really the asanas are much more than that. I've already given a list of what benefits the postures can give, such as balancing muscles, joints, glands, nerves and organs, as well as reducing fatigue and helping to soothe and discipline the mind and keep the body free from disease. But the postures are not exercise in the way that we generally understand exercise – they are not something that should cause you great exertion or strain. Unlike most forms of exercise, yoga is non-competitive – you work at your own pace without worrying about how more advanced anyone else may be.

One of the first things yoga postures do is to stretch everything, and stretching is amazingly beneficial: it relieves tiredness and tension, loosens tight muscles and encourages the release of endorphins – the body's natural tranquillizer.

Yoga postures are always practised in conjunction with your breathing – for example, you breathe in as you lift a limb, and out as you lower it. In this way, you learn to do things more slowly, in rhythm with your breath. You will gain better breath control and learn better body awareness as you learn to co-ordinate your movements.

When you learn the yoga postures you will also learn how to relax properly in the Pose of Complete Rest, which I explained in the last chapter. It is said that this posture is the most difficult to learn, because most of us find it very difficult to let everything go! Don't ever feel guilty about practising relaxation. Yoga is about *who* you are – and not about what you *do*. So do give yourself time to relax after a yoga session – and between the postures if you need to. Relaxation will help recharge your batteries and release new energy. It will overcome any exhaustion brought about by stress. It also clears blockages at a deep level so healing can take place. I have witnessed how relaxation can undo tension on several occasions, when people have broken down and cried during a yoga relaxation class. This is because they had been holding on to tension and grief for many years, and the relaxation then started to unblock their energy centres and release stress so they could experience their true emotions again. I'm not suggesting that when you practise the relaxation exercise you will break down, but the release of feelings can start to put you back in control of yourself again. Yoga *will* help you to bring about peace of mind. As years of tension start to shift you will find yourself able to listen in more and able to take control – and you will discover much more energy! This will take practice – most of us go through our lives not even aware that we *are* tense much of the time. It's only by practising relaxation every day that you will start to realize the difference between being tense and being relaxed. However, once you have gained this awareness, you can use it outside your yoga session, so that if anything does make you stressed, you can consciously relax.

The Pose of Complete Rest
Lie down on the floor or on your bed with your eyes closed. Keep your legs slightly apart and your palms facing upwards. Wriggle your heels down so that your feet fall away from your hips and relax apart. Wriggle your hands down to lengthen the space between your neck and shoulders. Now take yourself through each part of your body, tensing each muscle group then relaxing. Start with your feet, tense all the muscles in your toes, feet and ankles, then relax them. Now squeeze the muscles in your legs – your calf and thigh muscles – as tightly as possible and lift your legs up slightly from your support. Hold for a few seconds then relax. Pull your tummy muscles in, then relax. Hold your arms out and make fists with your hands, then relax them. Lift your shoulders up towards your ears, then relax them downwards. Think about any tension in your back and shoulders and allow it to ease away as you sink into your support. Now squeeze your face together as tightly as possible, then relax. Feel your jaw relax and the space between your eyebrows ease, and imagine someone is massaging your scalp so that all the tension in your face and head disappears. Try to relax your whole body as much as possible. Feel your whole body grow heavy as it sinks into your support – there is no need for you to hold on to any tension at all. Pay particular attention to your jaw,

shoulders, back and stomach – the areas where you carry most of your stress.

I would suggest that you try to practise the Pose of Complete Rest every day. When you stretch a muscle this it helps it to relax more when you let it go, although eventually you will be able to do the relaxation sequence without having to tense your muscles first. If you don't have much time, do this pose before you go to sleep. As you practise more, you will start to learn how your body feels when it is relaxed compared to how it feels when tense. You can then carry this awareness with you into everyday situations so that if you *are* under stress, you can consciously drop your shoulders, unlock your jaw and slow down your breathing. This is a very powerful tool to help you cope with tension, which causes fatigue.

Pranayama – The Control of Energy through Yoga Breathing

Pranayama is the fourth limb of yoga. Prana, as already discussed, means universal energy or life force, and pranayama is the process of directing into and controlling and storing this energy in the body using yoga breathing techniques. The word pranayama actually means control of prana or life-force energy.

As I said in the section on hyperventilation in Chapter 1, how you breathe profoundly affects your health and emotions. For example, if you are angry or tense, you will probably breathe rapidly from the upper part of your chest area, which means you won't be using your diaphragm. This also works the other way round – in other words, if under normal circumstances you breathe quite fast and only from your chest, this will eventually affect your thoughts and emotions. You may become agitated, depressed and anxious, because your body is not receiving the correct combination of oxygen and carbon dioxide. Your concentration may slow down. And of course this will make you very fatigued. It is said in yoga that one outburst of anger uses up three month's supply of energy! If you are constantly under pressure, shallow breathing may become your normal way of life, even when the stress has passed. Because your state of mind is controlled by the way you breathe, it stands to reason that you can reverse this process and control your mind by taking control of your breathing. Most of us don't take much notice of how we breathe – it is an unconscious action. Pranayama exercises will show you how to become more aware of this.

Taking control of your breathing can lead to a state of deep calmness. It is said in yoga that we are allotted only a certain number of breaths in life – so a person with rapid, shallow breathing may live a shorter life than someone who breathes slowly and deeply. Proper breathing cleanses the system, refreshes and invigorates the mind, increases alertness and concentration, and can renew the subtle energy body (your aura) so that healing can happen. It helps promote deeper sleep, relieves tension, improves the digestion, lowers blood pressure, slows the heartbeat and generally leads to a more contented state of being. That's a lot of reasons to make pranayama part of your everyday routine!

Breathing Exercise
Lie on the floor or on the bed, on your back. First of all, tune in to your breathing rhythm. Is your breathing fast or slow? Try to slow it down so that you breathe in for a count of four, then out to a count of four. This is one cycle. Using a clock or watch with a minute hand, time yourself and try to do around 12 cycles a minute. (Although this is the rate to aim for, it is not important at this stage if your breathing rate is higher.) Now put your hands on your solar plexus (just above your navel.) Breathe in: you should feel the movement of your diaphragm as your lungs inflate and it swells into your abdominal cavity. Try and keep your abdomen firm at this point. Now move your hands one hand width up so they are on the lower part of your ribcage. Your whole ribcage should move up and down as you breathe, with your hands moving up and out as you breathe in, and

down as you breathe out. Let your diaphragm rise unrestricted as you breathe. To emphasize this action, put your hands around your ribcage with your thumbs to the back and your fingers to the front. As you breathe in, feel your ribcage expand upwards and outwards. Squeeze it in gently as you breathe out.

Start to get used to the difference between your in-breath and your out-breath, and try to develop an awareness of your diaphragm when you breathe, so that you never breathe just from your upper chest. Practise this twice a day for five minutes. – perhaps when you wake up and just before you go to sleep. As you get used to this way of breathing, incorporate it in your daily routine – whether you are sitting or standing. Check yourself several times a day. Are you still breathing using your diaphragm? Does your breathing need to be slower? If you are ever in a stressful situation – for example, if you are in confrontation with someone – consciously slow down your breathing. You will be amazed at how much calmer and in control you feel.

Meditation

There are many reasons why meditation, the seventh limb of yoga, is important. Meditation calms and heals the mind and gives a huge boost of energy that is as refreshing – if not more so – than sleep. And meditation can also help you to develop your spiritual awareness and find your own truth, the real you and your purpose in life. If you are not interested in your spiritual development and you are reading this book only to discover more energy, you will still find meditation an invaluable tool for fighting fatigue. Meditation is a state of mind where your brain rhythms actually slow down. This happens when you sit still, with your spine upright and your brain clear of all thoughts. It's rather like looking at a blank cinema screen – you still your mind and think of nothing. Howard Kent uses the analogy of a car engine: most of us are using the engine with a foot on the throttle, but when we meditate we take the foot off, and the engine – or mind – just ticks over.

Personally, I have experienced very deep peace and stillness through meditation, and it has enabled me to get through many crises, including the death of a close member of my family. It takes time and perseverance to learn, and you must be disciplined enough to make 20 minutes free for meditation every day – but the benefits are well worth the effort. There is more about how to meditate in Chapter 9.

THE YOGA DIET

In the last chapter you may have begun to realize that diet plays a vital role in energy production. If you are tired, stressed or suffering from a condition such as depression or hypoglycaemia, what you eat will affect you greatly. Most people don't realize that diet forms part of yoga. I've talked about prana or life-force energy, and in yoga eating the right food is one of the major ways to obtain this.

You may remember that in yoga you get your energy from the sun, air, soil and water. One of the most effective ways your body can get energy is from the metabolism of food. The storehouse for prana in your body is believed to be in your solar plexus (your navel area, where digestion takes place), so good food is vital for good health. Think of your food as medicine – if you want energy then you must eat food of quality. If you eat food of poor quality, you will feel fatigued and unwell. When you are tired, it is more tempting to eat quick, ready-prepared meals – but this is the time when you really need to pay more attention to your diet than ever before.

The first thing to understand is that food also has a vital energy force. In order to benefit from this food-energy, you have to eat food in as near to its natural state as possible. This is because food that has just been picked has much more prana. So whenever possible eat only whole foods that have not undergone processing in any way. Ideally, you should pick a home-grown vegetable and eat it on the spot! This isn't always possible, but food that has been stored too long on the supermarket shelf or in your fridge; food that has been sprayed with pesticides or treated with hormones and antibiotics; food that is overcooked or left over from the day before will not have any prana that your body can use. These processes destroy the potential of the food you eat and actually *deplete* rather than increase your energy. Your diet should therefore include organic whole grains and pulses, fresh fruit and vegetables, eggs, beans, live yoghurt, nuts and seeds.

In yoga it is believed that a pure diet purifies the mind, so the food you should choose should be simple, sweet-smelling, light, nutritious and easily digestible. If you do eat meat, try to find organic or free-range products. The stress an animal experiences in an abattoir is very prana depleting and its fear is passed on through stress hormones in its meat. If you are going to follow the path of yoga strictly, you might choose not to eat meat at all, as this is contrary to the guidance given in the first limb of yoga (yama) which advises non-harm to any living being. Another reason for not eating meat is that if you eat the flesh of any living being, you are gaining your prana second-hand (the animal got the energy first-hand from the soil).

So think about what you eat, rather than cooking prepackaged meat and vegetables that have been stored on a supermarket shelf. Try to eat organic foods in season. There is a reason for this. In the winter, root vegetables can help you get more energy from the earth at a time when you are getting less from the sun. Try to eat local produce that won't have been spoilt by travelling and storage. Eat three nutritious meals a day – including breakfast – and if you have snacks, make sure they are of good quality, such as seeds and nuts. Try to cut out all sugar and sweet foods, as these will ultimately make you feel more fatigued. Drink alcohol in moderation – and if you have candida or hypoglycaemia, avoid it altogether. Do not embark on a calorie-controlled diet – this will seriously curtail your nutritional and energy intake. If you are eating proper nutritious food, you don't need to diet. As you practise yoga, you will eventually attain your ideal weight.

Preferred foods

In yoga the foods you should eat are known as Sattivic, which means food that is easy to digest, that gives lots of energy, and that helps to purify the system and calm the mind. Try to include as much of the following in your diet:

- organic fruit and vegetables grown locally and in season
- whole grains such as brown rice and sprouted wheat
- pulses such as chickpeas, soya beans and lentils
- seeds such as sunflower, pumpkin and sesame
- fresh nuts (not peanuts)
- milk (used traditionally in yoga as a source of protein)
- plain live yoghurt
- honey as a sweetener
- bottled or filtered water
- herbal teas

If all this sounds too difficult remember that yoga is about following the middle path – in other words, not doing anything that's too extreme. However, you do need to work towards a basic healthy diet before you can allow yourself the odd treat!

Finally, in yoga it is believed that much of the prana in food is absorbed through the tongue. So chew your food very thoroughly before you swallow – it should be like a fine paste. This will also help with your digestion: the nutrients are more easily absorbed into the bloodstream so you're less likely to develop food intolerances and won't use up so much energy digesting your food. Relax and sit down when you eat – we saw in the last chapter how stress leads to poor digestion because the digestive process slows right down when you are under pressure. Try not to drink water when you eat, as this will dilute the digestive juices. Eat only when you are hungry, and then only in moderation. Ideally, if you are eating good food which has been grown in soil of reasonable quality, you shouldn't need to take supplements. However, if you are suffering from fatigue it is possible that your digestive tract is not absorbing all the nutrients, especially if you suffer from candida. You could try taking vitamin C, a B vitamin complex, calcium and magnesium and evening primrose oil. Because we all have individual requirements, you may like to consider visiting a nutritional therapist for more advice.

Water

You've probably heard this before – you need to drink lots of water! Your body needs lots of lubrication so that everything can function – from circulation and elimination through to the working of all your organs. A yoga teacher cited the analogy of a car battery to me – unless your car battery is topped up with purified water, the engine won't function. So it is with your body – if you don't drink between $2^3/_4$ and $3^1/_2$ pints ($1^1/_2$ and 2 litres) of water a day, your body will not function as it should and you will feel fatigued.

WHAT YOGA REALLY MEANS

I hope this chapter has given you an idea of how yoga can help you. The word 'yoga' means to unite, and this is what yoga is about – helping us to unite with the infinite, or universe. In yoga, we are seen as having a real self – which is hidden away under our wants and desires. If you can rediscover your real self this will help you to experience your connection to everything in the universe, which will give you tremendous energy. Yoga isn't a religion, but it *is* a philosophy – a way of life that can help you discover your own path to health and vitality.

3

Energy and Your Energy Centres

In this chapter I'm going to talk about energy or prana in more detail, and show how working with it is fundamental to your vitality and health. If you understand prana, you will be able to make better use of it, particularly if you use the yoga breathing techniques (pranayama) in the next chapter.

PRANA – THE UNIVERSAL ENERGY FORCE

In the Introduction, I said that prana is a kind of cosmic energy and is thought to be the sum of all the energy in the universe. The ancient yogis said that this energy has no chemical or physical form, but is our true nourishment. We take prana into our bodies via the nadis, subtle energy channels which feed our chakras or energy centres. I shall explain nadis and chakras in more detail later on, but for now I want to try and give you a better idea of what prana is. Interestingly, since the ancient yogis of India discovered and worked with prana, science in the 20th century is now coming to the same conclusion – that there *is* some form of Universal Energy Force!

Let's compare a couple of views on this. The writer Andre van Lysebeth proposes that prana may be electromagnetic, or at least composed partly of electrically charged particles. Following this theory through, he suggests that certain locations – such as mountainous regions and the seaside – have more prana because they are highly charged with negative ions. To me this makes sense – I certainly feel invigorated when I am skiing or near the sea. Howard Kent from the Yoga for Health Foundation says: 'The constituent parts of prana are not yet wholly understood, but clearly include oxygen, the electromagnetic force and probably negative and positive ions.' These two yoga experts agree that prana includes *all* forces of nature known to man, including gravity, light, heat, electricity, magnetism, the nervous system and the mind.

In quantum physics, everything that exists in the universe is seen as having patterns of energy – of which atoms are a part. For example, as you may know, if two atoms merge they have incredible energy – enough to power a small town. I am not talking about fusing or splitting atoms here; I use this only as an example to show how much energy exists in even the smallest particle in the universe, and to explain that these particles are in constant motion – that is, they are moving in patterns of energy.

The Theory of Relativity shows that mass has nothing to do with a substance, but is a form of energy. So every tiny particle in the universe is *not* a static object but a process involving energy, which manifests as the particle's mass. That includes you! Put simply, this means that you – and every object you can think of – are a mass of vibrating bits of energetic particles. This is quite amazing if you think about it! It's even more incredible if you understand that you can learn how to *use* this tremendous energy through yoga! Three hundred years ago, the physicist Sir Isaac Newton saw all these particles as separate, and it is only recently that science has discovered that all matter is interconnected, interrelated and interdependent. At the beginning of the 20th century for example, the physicist Niels Bohr showed that all particles in the universe are constantly 'in touch' with each other – informing one another of what is happening. So particles are actually entangled, forming a huge cosmic web of interacting particles. This brings us on to the unity I talked about in Chapter 2, when I said that the aim of yoga is to help us to realize that we are *not* separate, but united and part of everything. Because all particles in the universe are connected and related, each one influences everything else. It is said that if a butterfly flaps its wings, the effect will be felt on the most distant star. So imagine how *your* actions affect everything in the universe!

What I am saying is that our universe *does* have a unity – of which we are part – and it also has energy, even if it *seems* to be an inanimate mass. This energy is prana – and prana is our link to the universe. By using yoga techniques, prana can be controlled, directed and stored at will. If you can learn to tap in to prana, you can have access to limitless energy! You will learn some of these techniques when we look at the special breathing techniques in Chapter 4, but meanwhile here are some suggestions to help you maximize on prana, the universal energy force.

- Try to walk barefoot on the ground at least once a day to benefit from the earth's natural electric field. Recent scientific research has found that we may have a sixth sense which responds to the earth's magnetic field; an organ which detects changes in geomagnetic fields has been found in fish, and it is thought humans may have this too. Renewing contact with the earth is particularly important if you have been travelling – cars, trains and aeroplanes act as a Faraday cage (an environment which prevents electromagnetic energy from passing through) and consequently block out the earth's natural prana. This is one reason why travelling can be so tiring.
- If possible, don't spend too much time in buildings or structures made of metal.
- Try to avoid air conditioning, smoke, dust and pollution. These are enemies of prana. If you live in a town, try to spend as much time in the country as you can. I know this isn't always possible, but at least be aware of your environment.
- Sunbathe when possible to increase your intake of solar prana. As with all things in yoga, do this in moderation.
- Take as much fresh air as possible. Use an ionizer in your

home if you can, especially if you live with anyone who
smokes.
- Avoid using plastic or synthetic materials; they attract
positive ions and reduce prana. Try to store food in paper or
glass, and try to wear only natural fibres such as cotton or silk.
- Most important of all, remember that prana is raised by
positive thinking – especially if you direct it with awareness –
because the mind is in part prana. The guided visualizations
in the next section on chakras will help you do this.
- Finally, yoga postures, good food, sunlight, fresh air, correct
breathing techniques and meditation can all encourage prana
to flow.

Now we shall look at nadis, the channels which enable you to
take in prana from the universe to feed your chakras and your
whole system.

NADIS – YOUR ENERGY CHANNELS

The word 'nadi' means a channel or tube. Nadis are the
conductors of prana; in other words, they are channels for
the circulation of vital energy. There are said to be at least 72,000
nadis that are related to our body. Some yoga experts have said
that nadis are like our nerves, but others disagree. The best way
to explain is to say that nadis are very similar to the subtle
energy channels known as meridians in Chinese medicine. I like
to think of nadis as electric currents that enable prana to be taken
in from the universe, giving energy to the material body. In a
radio set analogy, prana would be the radio waves and our
chakras the aerials that pick them up and circulate them round
the body via the nadis.

Practising yoga helps to keep the nadis open, so that maximum
energy or prana can flow. Certain yoga breathing techniques do
this very effectively and are very energizing. For example,
Alternate Nostril Breathing in Chapter 4 works on the major
nadis, and this in turn helps to purify the whole network of nadis.

The three major nadis that I want to talk about relate to the spine and nostrils. I have explained that we have our own electromagnetic field, and it is important that you know that yoga has always recognized this kind of energy, long before electricity was discovered. For example, in yoga, polarity – or negative and positive – is a very important concept because it involves the *balance* of the complete whole. The physical postures in yoga are sometimes referred to as Hatha yoga. 'Hatha' means sun (ha) and moon (tha) – in other words, it incorporates the two opposite ideas of day and night. In yoga it is believed that the left nostril carries the nadi which is the moon, or feminine energy which relates to the negative pole. The right nostril carries the nadi which is the sun, or masculine, positive energy. They intertwine and descend along the spine, the main nadi. This is why the spine is so important in yoga, because it carries vital energy to feed the main chakras. So good posture really will help your energy levels.

THE CHAKRAS – YOUR ENERGY CENTRES

As we have already seen, yoga understands prana as the basic source of life energy, and the body takes in energy via nadis to a series of centres called chakras. Understanding your chakras will help you to understand and explore your own energy. There are many chakras in the body, but I will concentrate on the main seven, which run parallel with the spine (*see* figure 3). These chakras vibrate with a particular frequency, which also relates to sound and colour. If your energy becomes blocked and a chakra is not vibrating as it should, you become out of balance and ill health and fatigue will follow.

In Sanskrit, chakra means a wheel or vortex – and that is what a chakra is, a spinning vortex which takes in energy to feed all areas of the human system: your physical and your subtle body. Chakras work on a physical, emotional and spiritual level and, as we shall see, each one relates to a particular area of the body. Although I will be talking about each chakra separately later on, it's important

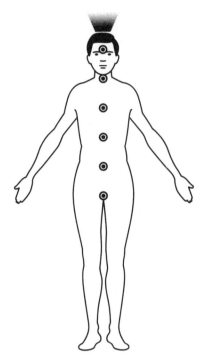

Crown Chakra – Ultra violet

Brow Chakra – Midnight blue

Throat Chakra – Light blue

Heart Chakra – Green

Solar Plexus Chakra – Yellow

Sacral Chakra – Orange

Base Chakra – Red

Figure 3   The chakras

to understand that they are all related. We can't really understand our individual chakras without looking at all of them. At the end of this chapter I will give you two exercises to help balance *all* your chakras. The chakras have Sanskrit names but to make things simple I shall refer to them by their English names. The seven main chakras are as follows, with the first five all located along the spine.

- The Root or Base Chakra, at the bottom of the spine, with the funnel pointing downwards to bring up energy from the earth
- The Sacral Chakra, between the pubic bone and the navel
- The Solar Plexus Chakra, located at the navel
- The Heart Chakra, just to the right of the heart
- The Throat Chakra, at the throat
- The Brow Chakra, just above the point between the eyebrows

- The Crown Chakra, just above the top of the head, with the funnel pointing upwards to take in energy from above

Your chakras are like energy stepping stones – as you work up to your higher energy centres towards the Crown Chakra, the vibration rate increases. You may remember that when I was explaining prana I said every particle and atom in the universe vibrates with energy. This vibration happens at different frequencies – for example, light has a much higher electromagnetic vibration than sound. So each chakra vibrates and each chakra transmits energy from one level to another, distributing pranic energy to the physical body. The lower chakras relate to your more earth-bound, emotional states and the higher ones to your spiritual state.

Your chakras can exist in two states: open or blocked. They can also become closed, but that only happens when you die. To put it simply, just remember that if your chakra is blocked it is taking in less prana and if it is too open it may be taking in more energy than you are able to cope with. As an example, after a bereavement, grief may open your Heart Chakra too quickly to passionate emotions, which may be overwhelming. On the other hand, if you try to ignore the feelings of grief and deny your emotions, you will eventually block the energy of the Heart Chakra. Blocked chakras can lead to distorted thinking and perception, anger and neurosis, or the over-use of defence mechanisms such as repression and being out of touch with your feelings. This eventually leads to physical ailments that relate to the specific chakras. It is important, therefore, that as you listen in more to yourself using yoga, you learn the lessons your chakras show you and don't try to block any emotional pain or experience. Otherwise you will become ill: losing your energy may be the first clue that this is happening.

I'm now going to talk about each chakra in more detail so that you will have a better idea of which particular area *you* need to work on. As I've indicated, each chakra relates to a colour, emotion and physical area of your body. The first four also have related elements. I'll also explain what can happen if the chakra is too open or closed. At the end of each section there are exercises for you to try. Details of specific yoga postures which will help you to work on each chakra are given in Chapters 5–8.

The Root or Base Chakra

- At the physical level your Root Chakra relates to your adrenal system, your lower bowel and your system of elimination.
- The Root chakra vibrates as the colour red. It is represented by the element of earth and consequently has a solid, dense frequency.
- Emotionally, the Root is your anchor and foundation chakra. It is about being in the real material world, being grounded in the here and now. It is also associated with the will to live and *wanting* to be alive – the sense of 'I am here!'
- A blocked Root Chakra can leave you lacking in energy, with a weak constitution and a feeling of being depersonalized. You may feel you are not really here, you may live in your head too much, or you may indulge in excessive daydreaming. It can also lead to a fear of letting go and opening up to your inner creativity. Having a blocked Root Chakra can be likened to a tent with insecurely attached guy ropes, making the structure unsound.
- If your Root Chakra is too open, you may be so grounded in the 'here and now' that you lose touch with your spiritual horizons and become very materialistic.
- If the Root Chakra is balanced you will be able to accept yourself, your body and your life as they are and consequently enjoy a feeling of security, confidence and self-esteem. Your energy and enthusiasm for life emanate from this chakra when it is vibrating correctly.

Susie's Story
I worked in a large library of a university and was also researching for my PhD. I always used to put a lot of pressure on myself to work

hard – and I suppose I am quite cerebral; I would rather read a book than play a game of tennis! About three years ago I had a nervous breakdown. It started with panic attacks – I would wake up in the middle of the night unable to breathe or swallow, with my heart pounding so fast that I thought I was going to have a heart attack. I also would feel very faint and, most frightening of all, I felt very unreal, as if I wasn't really there. I was tired all the time – so exhausted in fact that I could hardly work. I grew more and more afraid – of what I don't really know, but everything made me so fearful that I became suicidal. I lost all my confidence and thought I was a terrible person – a complete failure. I felt as if my whole life was slipping out of my control and I physically tensed my whole body to try to hold on. My doctor prescribed Valium and antidepressants which just made me more tired. To cut a long story short, I got worse and couldn't leave my house without panicking. I was referred to a private psychiatric hospital. I thought it would be terrible there but it was brilliant. They had a yoga class every day, which I joined – and to my amazement I started to feel better, more *here*, if you know what I mean. The yoga teacher taught me some breathing techniques and explained how to control my breathing so that I didn't hyperventilate. She suggested that I could do some work on my Root Chakra and showed me how to ground myself using visualization. I also took up pottery in hospital – and gardening, which I found very soothing. When I was well enough I was discharged from hospital, and I then decided to put my research work on hold while I retrained as a landscape gardener. I now spend lots of time working outside. I also do about half an hour of yoga every day and I belong to a group which I go to once a week. Yoga has helped to ground me; it made me realize that there are more important things in life than getting qualifications – but best of all it has given me boundless energy!

Exercises to Balance the Root Chakra

The Root Chakra faces downwards from the base of the spine to take in energy from the earth. These suggestions are to help you get back in touch with yourself using this energy, and for this reason they include visualization but not meditation. Meditation is excellent for balancing the upper chakras, but if you think your Root Chakra is blocked, leave meditation until you feel more grounded. Remember, it is vital for the health of all your chakras to have the Root Chakra balanced. Like a tree, the deeper your roots, the further your branches can reach out to the sunlight.

Visualization
Sit cross-legged so that your spine is in contact with the floor. Close your eyes and visualize a ray of red light coming up through the floor into your spine on an in-breath. On the out-breath, breathe the colour into your whole body so that you are bathed in a red energizing light. Really think about the colour. Imagine what it might smell and taste like. Imagine that you have become the colour red. Now look around the room. Be aware of everything in the room. Look at the ceiling and the walls and the furniture. Notice any ornaments, objects or books. Feel the texture of this book that you are holding. Listen for any sounds. Can you smell anything in the room? Rub your hands together and be aware of yourself in the room. Now stand up, keeping your back as straight as possible, your shoulders relaxed and your head lifted. Imagine red roots going down from your feet into the floor and through into the ground, taking in nourishment and energy from the earth.

Yoga Postures
To select postures for the Root Chakra, you need to look at anything that gets the base of the spine in contact with the ground. Try the Sitting Forward Stretch, the Boat and the Sitting Twist, which you will find in Chapters 5–8. The Pose of Complete Rest is also excellent for this chakra.

Other ways
Anything that gets you in contact with the earth or helps you to be in the 'here and now' of the material world is beneficial.

Walking, gardening, dancing or creative pursuits such as pottery are all excellent. Try walking barefoot across the grass – or just sitting in the garden appreciating the beauty of nature and the wonder of creation. You can also try wearing red clothes – such as socks, trousers or skirts – below the waist (ie near the Root Chakra).

The Sacral Chakra

- The Sacral Chakra is associated with the reproductive system, including the ovaries and uterus, the testes and the prostate. It is also responsible for the bladder and kidneys. Infertility, vaginal and pelvic infections, premenstrual syndrome (PMS), endometriosis, male infertility, impotence or prostatic diseases may indicate that this chakra is out of balance. Many of these can also cause fatigue.
- This chakra is represented by the element of water and the colour orange.
- At an emotional level, the Sacral Chakra is about the creation of life; it also relates to your sensual side and how you convey this to others. Therefore if this chakra is blocked it may show as a disruption in sexual relations with your partner.
- A Sacral Chakra that is too open can lead to envy, lust, fear, confusion or over-dependence on your partner.
- The Sacral Chakra is also concerned with the balance between female and male – yin (female) and yang (male) in Chinese philosophy, or Ha Tha in Sanskrit. Therefore when the Sacral Chakra is balanced, you can be independent and whole *and* contribute to the balance within an interdependent relationship.

Exercises to Balance the Sacral Chakra

Visualization
Lie on the floor and relax everything as much as possible. Close your eyes and imagine you are walking barefoot through a

wood. Smell the fragrant, energizing scent of the pine trees in the forest and of the woodland flowers that grow next to the path. Feel the texture of the wood mulch under your feet. In the distance you can hear a stream babbling. Walk towards the sound. You see a fast running brook filled with amber water. Imagine you are cupping your hands together and filling them with the golden liquid. Hold the water to your mouth and drink it. Feel the colour amber lighting up your whole body and giving you energy as you drink the liquid. Now walk downstream. You come across a large pond, where the water has been dammed. The water looks mysterious and deep – but inviting. You take off all your clothes and immerse yourself in the warm water. Imagine you are lying on your back for a while and just floating as the water soothes, purifies and caresses you. When you get out of the water, tell yourself you are now refreshed and revitalized.

Yoga Postures
Yoga postures for the Sacral Chakra include pelvic exercises such as the Pelvic Tilt. Other excellent postures are the Cat and the Locust.

The Solar Plexus Chakra

- At the physical level your Solar Plexus Chakra relates to your pancreas, stomach, liver, gall bladder, spleen and your small intestine. Eating disorders, hypoglycaemia, diabetes, pancreatic problems, indigestion and irritable bowel syndrome may be associated with this chakra being unbalanced.
- The Solar Plexus Chakra is represented by the element of fire and the colour yellow.
- Your Solar Plexus Chakra is your true energy centre, also known as your inner fire or sun centre. One of the reasons for this is that you get your stamina by the process of digesting

food. This is why the right food is considered *very* important in yoga, because it provides the energy for maintaining life – and can certainly help you to beat fatigue!

- Your Solar Plexus Chakra is also the centre for your major emotions, your ambitions, your wants and desires. It is your ego centre. If the Root Chakra is where you are grounded in the physical world and the sense of 'to be', your Solar Plexus Chakra is your centre of 'I am'. From this comes the expression that someone is very 'centred', referring to how they are in relation to other people. One of the most energy depleting experiences is living your life through others and experiencing other people's emotions, rather than having clear boundaries between yourself and those around you.

- If this chakra is too open it can act as an antenna that may pick up the negative energy of others too quickly. You may also be over-emotional, greedy, angry or aggressive. Or you may become a 'people pleaser', always thinking of other people's feelings but never looking after your own needs properly. This can make you overly submissive, passive and powerless, which can lead to resentment and real exhaustion.

- If your Solar Plexus Chakra is too closed, you may have the opposite experience and become selfish and unfeeling. Lack of drive and will power, an inability to project yourself in the world, depression, exhaustion and stress are all associated with a blocked Solar Plexus.

- For a healthy Solar Plexus Chakra, you need to learn to separate your own emotions and responsibilities from other people's, and to be open to experiences and not block your feelings. When we looked at the section on stress we saw how stored emotions cause tension and exhaustion. Because this chakra relates to your emotions, often you can actually *feel* tension around this area if you have an emotional upset. For example, if you have a shock, you may have the physical feeling that you have been punched in the stomach. If something makes you frightened or anxious, you are probably going to have 'butterflies in your tummy'. When your Solar Plexus Chakra is balanced, you will feel centred and confident, and you will be flexible rather than rigid in your thinking. You will be able to show your emotions, but you will be in control of these emotions, rather than the other way around. This will give you tremendous confidence and energy.

Exercises to Balance the Solar Plexus Chakra

Visualizations

1 If you feel that other people drain you, try imagining a mirror placed between you and them. Any negative energy they give out is therefore reflected back to them, rather than absorbed by you. And any positive energy that you give out is reflected back to you so that they are unable to drain off your vitality. Another excellent visualization is to imagine a white light surrounding you. This will protect you from negative energies.

2 This is a real energy-boosting visualization. Lie on the floor and relax as much as possible. Now breathe in and out slowly from your ribcage area, using your diaphragm. Try and slow down your breathing. Now imagine that you can feel the sun warming your abdomen. Imagine that you are breathing the golden globe of the sun into your sun centre – your Solar Plexus Chakra. Feel this warm golden light emanating from this centre, filling the rest of your body with yellow-gold energy and vitality.

Yoga Postures

The Bow and the Boat are good postures for balancing the Solar Plexus Chakra. One of the most beneficial postures in yoga for dealing with negative emotions, particularly anger, is the Woodchopper.

The Heart Chakra

- At the physical level, your Heart Chakra relates to your blood and circulation, your heart, lungs and your thymus gland. Because of its association with the thymus gland a blocked Heart Chakra can lead to problems with your immune function – or even, not surprisingly, heart problems.
- The Heart Chakra is represented by the colour green and the element of air.
- Your emotions rise from your Solar Plexus Chakra to your Heart Chakra, where they are translated into the higher feelings of love, harmony and compassion. This includes love and openness for yourself as well as for others. Unconditional love flows through this chakra – for mankind and all living beings – and helps you to see only the good in others.
- If your Heart Chakra is too open you may be too sensitive and over-concerned with others' needs. All your love and compassion will flow out towards others, which will make you very exhausted.
- If this chakra is blocked you may have a problem in maintaining loving relationships. For example, you might see others as hostile and threatening, rather than kind and giving. If you ever think that you are cold, or ruthless and detached from others or from your own feelings, you probably need to do some work with this chakra.
- As with all your chakras, your Heart Chakra needs to be balanced so that your energy can flow; if you are over-emotional or have difficulty showing your emotions, you will feel fatigued and physically drained because this energy is blocked.

Emma's Story
I've always had difficulty in expressing my emotions. As a child I was always told not to cry and that it was wrong to complain about anything. I suppose in the end I became very detached from everything – I even remember not being able to cry when

my mother died. I used to feel as if I was acting a role in life, somehow not really connected to anything. I was very ambitious and worked my way up to Head of Personnel in a large retail company. I married and had two children. Of course I loved them, but I found it very difficult to show them any real affection – I was never one to cuddle or touch a lot. I found trying to hold down my job and run a family unbelievably tiring. My husband works abroad a lot so I was in a way like a single parent, trying to work hard and deal with the children on my own. The house was always in a mess and inevitably backup support such as part-time nannies and cleaners let me down. I suppose I resented my life, but at the time I never actually stopped to question how *I* felt – I was too busy trying to run everything smoothly for everyone else and work hard to pay our huge mortgage. I was Super Woman, in charge of everything – from organizing school runs, managing the house and doing the shopping and cooking, to holding down a full-time job. I used to joke that the only time I had to myself was in the car on the way to work or in the bathroom! In the end I felt like a wrung-out dishcloth with absolutely *no* spark of energy – I was just getting through every day as best I could. I joined an aerobics class to see if I could get more energy, but that just became something else on my list I that had to fit in. I started having problems at work; my manager was always getting at me and made an official complaint that I was cold and unfeeling towards those whom I dealt with. I was so run down that I got ill with really bad angina attacks, but this turned out to be a blessing in disguise because it slowed me down and made me start to assess what I wanted in life. I took a month off work, and my husband and I decided to move to a smaller house so that I could work part-time. I then joined a yoga class, which was a real turning point. I started to meditate every day and really enjoyed the sense of calm it gave me. Meditation helped me to connect with my real self at last. I thought of meditation as my time, my 'treat'; it was never another thing on a list to do. My yoga teacher suggested that I should keep a 'feelings' diary, which I did. At first it was hard to know how I really did feel, but over the months, as I started to write, it just all flowed out of me – how I felt unwanted as a child, how I used to resent my husband and children and colleagues at work. I felt purged, really cleansed, and I was able to cry for the first time in years. I'm now so much happier and I have incredible energy – not just because I gave up working full-time, but because yoga helped me to release all the emotional tension I had held on to for years.

Exercises to Balance the Heart Chakra

Yoga Postures
Any posture that helps open up the chest area is beneficial for the Heart Chakra. Backward bends are therefore very good. Try the Cobra, where the hand position is near your chest. Also try the Fish and the Head of a Cow.

Other Ways
Whenever possible try surrounding yourself with nature. The greenness in nature is very therapeutic and will help to lift your energies upwards. Try walking barefoot on the grass. Also touch and cuddle your loved ones as much as you can. Yoga helps you to tune in to your Heart Chakra and get in touch with your feelings.

Try closing your eyes and repeating the mantra 'My heart beats quietly and regularly with love.'

The Throat Chakra

- At the physical level, your Throat Chakra is related to your thyroid gland, your vocal cords, your ears and the endocrine system. Breathing problems such as hyperventilation, asthma, emphysema and bronchitis may indicate that the Throat Chakra is unbalanced. Other clues that this chakra needs working on include hypothyroidism, throat problems in general, mouth ulcers and hearing problems.

- The Throat Chakra is represented by the colour blue.
- This chakra is particularly concerned with how you communicate and express yourself in the world. A balanced Throat Chakra will help you to put forward your feelings and ideas, and this in turn can lead to an understanding of your true path in life.
- If your Throat Chakra is blocked you may find you have problems with words. People who speak very quietly or who are inarticulate may have a blocked Throat Chakra. If you suspect that you come across as cynical, hostile or sarcastic, this is another sign that you need to work on your Throat chakra. If you do sometimes express yourself in a negative way it is probably true to say that you are hiding your real self, partly because you lack confidence. In other words, this chakra may be blocked because, at another level, you are covering up with a false identity. This will make you very fatigued, even if you are unaware of this at a conscious level; trying to be someone that you are not is very tiring. Remember too, that how you verbalize your ideas and feelings helps to create your own reality – but negativity can actually create fatigue!
- If your Throat Chakra is too open you may be over-talkative without being truly analytical, and you may dominate conversations without saying anything of value. Again, this is very exhausting, both for you and for others. Talking too much can be a defence mechanism that helps you to avoid looking inwards and instead fills your life with trivia.
- If your Throat Chakra is balanced you'll be able to interact with the world by talking, listening and reading – all of which help you to learn and express your true feelings clearly. If you are true to yourself and communicate your thoughts positively, you will start to realize and experience real energy – or prana.

Exercises to Balance the Throat Chakra

Yoga Postures
The Shoulder Stand, the Plough, the Bridge and the Fish are all excellent postures for energizing the Throat Chakra.

Other Ways
Singing and chanting are all beneficial therapies for the Throat Chakra. Chanting can heighten your awareness, aid meditation and help balance the higher chakras. The vibration of sound will help you to tune in to your true self and will really help you in your fight against fatigue. You can also try using the mantra Aum, which I will explain at the end of this chapter.

Also, try keeping a feelings diary or writing poetry, reading, learning a new skill, or painting. Practising pranayama or yoga breathing techniques is vital for all chakras, but has particular relevance for the Throat Chakra.

The Brow Chakra

- The Brow Chakra relates to your eyes, your lower brain and your nervous system (including the pituitary and the pineal glands that are relevant for your hormones, which are so often associated with fatigue, particularly if you are under stress). Your Brow Chakra is also responsible for your hypothalamus, often known as the Master Gland because it controls so many functions, including sleep, temperature control and your emotions. The hypothalamus is often implicated in cases of Chronic Fatigue Syndrome, because if it is not functioning properly, your general vitality and emotional wellbeing will be affected.
- This chakra is symbolized by the colour indigo blue.
- Your Brow Chakra is responsible for your imagination and concentration. As one of your higher chakras, it is also related to your finer emotions and spiritual status.

- If this chakra is blocked you may suffer from negative thinking, learning difficulties, poor concentration, headaches and mental fatigue. In extreme cases, this can lead to confused thinking or even psychosis – a lack of understanding between reality and fantasy.
- If this chakra is too open too soon, you may exercise anxiety about your spiritual progress – especially if you are not sufficiently grounded by your Root Chakra or centred by your Solar Plexus Chakra.
- When the Brow Chakra is balanced, your creative spirit will flow freely. The Brow Chakra is about using your intuition and creative force. Activation of this chakra also helps with visualization, which in effect is seeing with the mind's eye. Visualization is very useful as an aid to meditation, and a powerful tool for beating exhaustion.

Exercises to Balance the Brow Chakra

Visualization
This exercise, called Candle Gazing, is commonly used in yoga to aid concentration for those who are new to meditation. It is easy to do and very effective.

First, light a candle in a darkened room. Sit a few feet away – on the floor or on a chair – and look at the flame. Try to clear your mind of everything else. After a few minutes, close your eyes. You will find that you can still see the candle flame, even though your eyes are closed. This is called the negative after-image. Concentrate on this negative image of the flame. Try to keep your mind empty of everything but this image. When the image starts to fade, open your eyes and look at the candle again. Practise this with your eyes open and then closed for about five minutes, increasing the time as you become more comfortable with the meditation.

Think about how this exercise makes you feel. Notice any changes that happen as you practise this over the months.

Yoga Postures
The Pose of a Child, and the Standing Dog Stretch are excellent for the Brow Chakra.

Other Ways
If you suffer from mental fatigue, visualization, meditation and yoga breathing exercises will help. However, always make sure you ground yourself with your Root Chakra before and after practising any of the suggested exercises, by wriggling the base of your spine on the ground to connect yourself with the earth.

The Alternate Nostril breath, described in Chapter 4 is excellent for the Brow Chakra.

The Crown Chakra

- At the physical level, the Crown Chakra is responsible for your upper brain and, like the Brow Chakra, for your pituitary and pineal glands.
- It is represented by the colour violet, and also white which is the whole colour spectrum. The Crown Chakra is an amalgamation of all the other chakras; if all the chakras are harmonies of notes, the Crown Chakra can be said to be the whole melody.
- If your Crown Chakra is blocked, you may suffer from depression, and you may find it difficult to accept life as it is. You may feel imprisoned in your body, with no spiritual connection or direction from within. This will make you feel drained and exhausted.
- Conversely, if your Crown Chakra is too open, you may become too stuck in the spiritual world and be unable to relate to the real, physical here and now. This can bring about anxiety and fear.
- The Crown Chakra, if balanced, is about acceptance and peace as opposed to fear and despair. Because the Crown Chakra represents all our chakras together, it is concerned with

understanding the total pattern of life and why we are here. As I have explained, yoga is about union, which includes the coming together of mind, body and spirit. If you truly want to beat fatigue you have to pay attention to your spiritual self as well as your physical body.

Exercises to Balance the Crown Chakra

You can balance this chakra best through a disciplined practice of meditation. This will free you from the constant mental exhaustion which results from the hum of thinking in your head. Meditation helps to enhance the slower Alpha waves of your brain, and to harmonize the hypothalamus and endocrine system, all of which affect your energy levels; so at this level it can be seen that meditation is vital for increasing vitality. There is more on how to meditate in Chapter 9.

Visualization
1 Close your eyes and relax as much as possible. Now imagine that you are breathing in a beautiful, translucent violet light at the point between your eyebrows. As you breathe out, this becomes a white light, which you breathe out through your Crown Chakra, up to the sky. Practise this for a few minutes.
2 Shut your eyes and imagine above your head a closed up lotus flower with many petals – as many as one thousand. The petals slowly start to open and, as they do, sunlight streams down into your head. Imagine this light and energy going through your head and down through all your chakras, slowly filling them with light.

Yoga Postures
The Pose of a Rabbit or Hare is a good posture for the Crown Chakra. (Experienced yoga students can practise the Head Stand

every day; I have not covered this posture in this book as it is best learnt under supervision.)

Exercises to Balance all your Chakras

Although you can work on each chakra individually, it is also important to work on all of them together so that you can achieve real balance and bring health and vitality into your life. The following exercise will help you to do this.

Visualization

Sit on the floor with your legs crossed, or on the back of your heels if this is more comfortable. Sit upright and don't allow yourself to droop or sink into your hips. Keep your shoulders relaxed and down. Now imagine that the base of your spine has roots that go down through the floor into the ground, and that your head and the top of your spine are reaching upwards, into the sky. Only imagine this; although you are sitting upright your spine should be relaxed, not pulled. Now close your eyes. Breathe in then out, slowly, from your diaphragm. On the out-breath, imagine your breath going from the top of your head, down your spine and out into the ground. On the in-breath, breathe up through the base of your spine into the top of your head and out to the sky. Continue with this visualization, with your breath going up your spine on the in-breath and down on the out-breath. Always ground yourself by ending on an out-breath. Practise this for three minutes, or longer if you feel comfortable.

Chanting and Yoga Mantras

Chanting using a *mantra* (a single word or short phrase) helps to bring all your chakras into balance. First of all, make sure you won't be distracted and turn the phone off. Because you will be making some noise, you might like to chant your mantra when there is no one else around! Sit cross-legged on the floor or kneel and sit on the back of your heels – or on a chair if this is more comfortable. Try to sit upright without slouching so that your solar plexus area is not constricted. Now take a deep breath in from your diaphragm and open your mouth as wide as possible while you project as loud as you can the sound 'Aaaaah'. After a few seconds, slowly bring your lips into a circle so the sound becomes 'ooo'. For the final part of the breath, bring your lips together and finish by humming 'mmm'. This sound should last as long as your out-breath so you need some power in this breath to add to the vibration of the sound. The sound should move from the back of your throat to the front of your mouth. When you put the sequence together it should sound like Aum, or Om, and you should feel your whole body vibrate with the sound. This vibration stimulates your nerve endings and can help to heal and balance your whole system.

I hope that this chapter has given you an insight into your own chakras or energy centres and how they relate to your physical, mental and spiritual health and vitality. We are now going to move on to pranayama or breathing techniques, which will enable you to control, direct and store prana or Universal Life Energy.

4

The Secret of Energy Control

In the last chapter we looked at prana, the vital energy of the universe. In this chapter I will introduce you to pranayama, which will help you to control, store and direct this energy. If you practise the exercises given in this chapter, you will increase your vitality enormously.

PRANAYAMA – YOGA BREATHING EXERCISES

Briefly, prana can be controlled by using various yoga exercises, including the postures. However, one of the main ways to control it is to practise yoga breathing techniques, especially when combined with *bandhas*, which I will explain later. By controlling your breath you can help to control prana, and by learning to control this Universal Energy you can start to control your mind. This is possible because breathing helps to bring the mind under control; and because your emotions actually affect your breathing, you can therefore affect your emotional state by thinking about the way you breathe – and changing it! For example, if you are anxious or fearful, you breathe rapidly from your upper chest. This goes back to the 'fight or flight' syndrome that we looked at earlier. If you are really concentrating on something you may notice that your breathing rate drops, or you might even hold your breath. If you are relaxed, your breathing becomes slow and deep. So next time you are in a stressful situation, try to slow down your breathing rate and see what difference it makes.

Before we go on to the pranayama exercises, it is important that you get your normal breathing rate under control. Make sure that you are using your diaphragm and not breathing too rapidly. In Chapter 2 I asked you to lie down and isolate your ribs, then showed you how to use this area for breathing. Now I'd like you to try this again, but this time sitting upright in a chair, keeping your back straight. Put your hands around your ribcage so that your thumbs are pointing towards your back (*see* figure 4). This will help you feel your diaphragm, the dome-shaped muscle which I told you about before. Firstly, try to listen to your breathing and slow it down. Now balance it to an in-and-out rhythm. As you inhale, allow your ribcage to expand

Figure 4   Feeling your diaphragm

upwards, sideways, and into your back. As you slowly exhale, your hands should come closer together – you can gently squeeze your ribs together if you want to help this action. As your lower ribs move up and out with your in-breath, your diaphragm drops and stretches. When you breathe out, your diaphragm rises into a cone shape. Try breathing in through your nose for a count of four, and out for a count of four. This is one round.

What you are aiming to do is to breathe rhythmically, from your ribcage area, and to breathe no more than 12–15 rounds a minute. By doing this you are not over-breathing and you are using your diaphragm. This should influence your normal way of breathing, so do check yourself during the day to ensure that you are breathing *more slowly* and from your diaphragm, especially if you are in a stressful situation.

When you breathe in this way, your upper chest area may rise slightly, which is fine as long as you are not breathing just from this area. Incidentally, some yoga experts used to teach diaphragmatic breathing by getting students to breathe into their navel area, using a technique called the three-part or full breath. Nowadays, however, it is generally held to be better practice – and more effective for energy production – to use the ribcage area just above the navel. Your abdomen should remain firm.

General Guidelines

Now you have learned to breathe properly you are ready to learn the pranayama exercises, which I have divided into two sections. The first includes some basic routines which you can practise every day for about three months. Start with one or two every day, including perhaps the Kapalabhati Breath, which needs to be built up slowly. For the Alternate Nostril sequence, start with about one minute of practice and gradually increase to a maximum of 10.

When you feel happy that you are benefiting from these basic sequences, you can move on to the Breath Retention exercises. Eventually you can increase your pranayama practice from 10 up to a maximum of 20 minutes a day, choosing exercises that suit you from the selection I suggest. However, I would recommend that you do this only after you have done lots of practice.

If you can persuade someone to read these instructions to you as you do the exercises, all the better; otherwise, read the exercises slowly and I can assure you that you will soon get the idea.

Before you start pranayama, bear in mind the following points:

- Your breathing should be rhythmic and smooth, not forced or jerky. Keep it slow.
- How you think is absolutely vital. The movement of your mind affects prana, so you should always think positively, imagining prana or energy filling your body as you practise. When you are doing the exercises, concentrate only on your breathing, the rhythm, and the idea of prana. Try not to let your mind wander. Keep your eyes closed – this will help your concentration. All these exercises are healing because they awaken prana, helping your whole system to become more balanced.
- Everything in the universe is vibration or energy – and in all vibration there is rhythm. So try to pay attention to the rhythm of your breathing.
- Practise pranayama *after* your yoga postures, not before – and always on an empty stomach. In the morning before breakfast is a good time. When you've finished, lie down in the Pose of Complete Rest for about five minutes.
- Always practise with an upright spine. This keeps the main nadi or energy channel open and thus helps the flow of prana.
- Always breathe through your nose unless otherwise instructed. The hairs in your nostrils help to filter out impurities, germs, dust and pollution. Breathing through your nose also warms the air, which protects your lungs.
- Unless otherwise instructed, remember to keep your abdomen firm and don't allow it to balloon out. Firm means controlled – not rigid.

- A cycle consists of one inhalation and exhalation – with retention if indicated.
- If you feel tired or dizzy, stop! Check with your doctor first if you are suffering from heart or lung problems. Never strain and *never* try to hold your breath for too long.
- Always exhale first so that you start a round on an in-breath.
- And finally, if you feel any stress during the day, practise some pranayama exercises and visualize that you are breathing in peace and strength and breathing out negativity. You will be amazed at how effective this is!

Basic Pranayama Exercises

Kapalabhati

This is an excellent exercise to use at the beginning of pranayama because it cleanses the lungs and prepares them for the exercises to follow. It is incredibly invigorating and involves a dynamic out-breath in short bursts, followed by a slower inhalation. As long as you return to normal breathing afterwards, you will receive enormous benefit from Kapalabhati. This breath removes stale air from your lungs and brings about a rapid expulsion of carbon dioxide so that your blood becomes saturated with oxygen. This stimulates cellular (internal) breathing, which is particularly beneficial if you lead a sedentary life. Kapalabhati breathing will calm your nervous system, massage your digestive tract and, most importantly, literally 'irrigate' your brain! (Your brain will be filled with fresh blood which will stimulate the endocrine, pituitary and pineal glands. In this way the brain is washed in oxygen-rich blood and cleansed of stagnant or sluggish circulating blood.) Poor blood flow to the brain has been shown to be evident in cases of Chronic Fatigue Syndrome, so you can see why the Kapalabhati breathing is so incredibly energizing.

A word of caution – do not practise this exercise if you have serious eye or ear complaints, if you suffer from high or low blood pressure, a hiatus hernia, any lung disorder, or if you are pregnant. Build up this sequence slowly from one round of 10 breaths to a maximum of 120 breaths, or 10 rounds of 10 fast breaths, which would eventually be done in one minute. I would suggest you add a round of 10 breaths each week, going from 10 to 20, then 30, and so on until you reach 120.

Kapalabhati is very energizing, which is why I am including it here, but I have to add that it is best practised under supervision, so if you know of a friendly yoga teacher you may like to ask for some help.

Method

Sit with your spine upright and identify your diaphragm area around your lower ribcage, as I have shown you. Now, using your abdomen like a piston, contract the muscles sharply to cause a violent expulsion of air – as if someone has punched you. Next, you will have to breathe in to fill the vacuum created by your out-breath. This should be automatic – it's rather like sneezing with your mouth closed! Repeat this exercise rapidly for 10 breaths. This is one round of Kapalabhati. Relax for three breaths. In your second week of practice, add 10 more breaths (another round), then rest again. Gradually build up to 120 breaths a minute, as explained above. Remember, this exercise should not be practised for more than a minute in any one session.

If you are feeling tired during the day try practising Kapalabhati. It really does combat fatigue and drowsiness because toxins are dissolved and the brain is recharged. This breath also increases concentration, improves memory and stimulates the intellect. It is especially refreshing if you have been working at a computer or in an office. Because this is technically a hyperventilation exercise (in other words, it induces a rapid intake of oxygen), remember to return to normal breathing when you have finished.

Alternate Nostril Breathing
You may remember I explained that your body has three main nadis that help conduct your prana or life energy throughout the body. Two of these are located in the nostrils and are related to positive and negative energies. This means that in order to be healthy, these nadis need to be kept clear and in balance. alternate nostril breathing helps to clear these two main nadis and also encourages harmony between the left and right sides of the brain. Science now tells us that we use one side of our brain more than the other. For example, creative people such as artists tend to use the right side, whereas scientists and mathematicians favour their left side, which is used for more rational and logical thinking. Using alternate nostril breathing can help to balance both hemispheres of the brain.

Method
Place one hand in front of your face, resting your two middle fingers on the bridge of your nose so that you can use your thumb to block one nostril and your ring finger the other. Support your elbow with your other hand if necessary. If you get tired, swap hands. Start by exhaling through both nostrils. Then block your right nostril and inhale through the left to a slow count of four. Now block your left nostril and exhale through the right using the same rhythm of four. Then inhale through your right nostril, block it, and exhale through your left. This completes one round. Continue like this, concentrating on the rhythm and making sure that both the in- and out-breath are complete and even. Practise this for one minute to start with, then increase the time. Close your eyes to aid your concentration.

The Ha Breath
This breath uses a sweeping arm movement which helps to pump great energy into your body. It also helps to cleanse stale air from your lungs.

Method
Stand upright, keeping your spine straight. Breathe out. Now breathe in and lift your arms up over your head. Breathe out. Breathe in, bending your knees and taking your arms slightly behind your head. Now, as you breathe out, let your trunk flop forwards, let your arms swing in front of you and open your mouth and force the air out. As you do so say 'haaaa', sighing the air out. This out-breath should last for about five seconds. Hold your position, relaxing your arms, head and trunk down for a few seconds, and then repeat five times.

Traditional Yoga Breathing
This exercise is very calming, and very simple to do.

Method
Breathe in slowly for a count of four, then breath out slowly for a count of six. You can vary this rhythm to suit your natural breathing pattern – for example, you may like to breathe in for a count of six and out for a count of eight.

This completes the basic pranayama exercises, which you should practise every day for about three months. Then you can move on to the more advanced breath retention exercises. But first I will explain bandhas, a Sanskrit word meaning a lock or seal.

Bandhas

Bandhas are locks that you can use to increase the effectiveness of your breath retention exercises, because they help to seal in energy or prana. Bandha means to tie, control or lock, and the positions involve various muscular contractions which affect the circulation of your blood, your nerves and endocrine system. There are three main bandhas: the Chin Lock, the Abdomen Lock, and the Root Lock. I'm going to describe these exercises here so that you can try them. When you feel comfortable with them, you can use them where indicated in the next sequence of pranayama.

The Chin Lock

Inhale, then holding your breath, press your chin down firmly into your chest, between the collarbones. As you exhale, slowly lift your chin back to its normal position.

This position compresses and stimulates the thyroid gland – in fact, it does this so effectively that if you have an over-active thyroid, you must not use it. It is very beneficial if you are suffering from fatigue.

The Abdomen Lock

Inhale, then exhale and pull the abdomen up and back towards the spine.

The Root Lock

This involves contracting your anal sphincter muscles. Inhale, hold your breath and contract your anus. When you can't hold your breath any longer, exhale and relax your anus. Repeat twice. As you do this, focus you attention on the anus as you contract it, then imagine the point above this and contract that too. This lock tones up the lower bowel and the pelvic floor area. It prevents constipation and haemorrhoids and is good for balancing your Root Chakra.

Combined Lock

To combine these three locks, stand upright, breathe in and lower your chin to your chest. Hold your breath and pull the lower abdominal area up towards your spine and pull up your anal muscles. Breathe out slowly and release the locks.

The following sequences – which involve all the bandhas – were introduced to me by my current yoga teacher Margo Dixon. They are both excellent for increasing energy.

Imaginary Rowing

Sit on the floor, with your legs out straight. Now imagine that you are pulling on the oars of a boat. Lean forward, arms outstretched and exhale. As you start to inhale, pull on the imaginary oars as you start to lean back, pressing your chin into your chest and tightening your abdominal and anal muscles. Hold your breath then release, rowing forward as you breathe out. Repeat this sequence up to 10 times.

Pot Stirring

For a variation on the above, pretend you are stirring a giant pot. From the same position, hold your hands together with your arms outstretched. Now move your arms in a large circle in time with your breath. At the end of your in-breath your chin should be on your chest, with your anal and abdominal muscles tight. At the end of the out-breath you should be leaning forward, outstretched over your legs.

Mudras

As well as bandhas, there are also *mudras* – hand positions which help close the circuits of energy in your body and direct the breath. You may like to use a basic position known as *jnana mudra* when you are practising the next sequence of pranayama exercises. It is very simple – just touch the tip of your index finger with the tip of your thumb, then either rest your hands on your knees (palms up), or keep the rest of your fingers outstretched. As well as closing your energy circuit, this mudra is said to stop the energy leaking out of your extremities!

Pranayama – Breath Retention Exercises

In yoga it is thought that we are allocated a set number of breaths, so that life is measured in breaths rather than years. Therefore it is thought that slowing down your breath will help to increase your life span. In pranayama, as well as learning to slow down your breathing you can learn to hold or retain your breath. This can greatly increase your energy because your respiration affects the circulation of your blood and is a powerful tonic for the whole system. Holding your breath helps prana to flow because it stimulates cellular breathing by helping your cells to absorb oxygen and to evacuate carbon dioxide more effectively. In other words, it gives a better 'digestion' of inhaled air. Breath retention also stimulates the spleen and makes it expel large quantities of red corpuscles into the bloodstream. It also produces heat in your body and can even increase the activity of your brain, because fluids are circulated more efficiently.

I am now going to describe seven different breath retention exercises. Start by selecting a few every day and gradually build up to about 10 minutes' practice. You will further increase your energy if you use the bandhas. As a guide I suggest you use the Chin Lock when holding your breath after an inhalation, and the Abdomen and Root Locks when holding your breath after an exhalation, unless otherwise instructed.

1 To start with, take five ordinary in-and-out-breaths, then hold the last one for a few seconds, holding then releasing the Chin Lock. Listen in to your body as you do so. Then exhale slowly and smoothly, pushing the air out by contracting your ribcage muscles. Don't breathe out suddenly. In this way you are controlling the inhalation, retention and exhalation. Practise a round of six per session.
2 The next exercise combines breath retention with alternate nostril breathing. Using the hand positions I showed you, block your right nostril and exhale slowly through your left nostril for a count of four seconds. Inhale through the left nostril then hold your breath for four seconds by blocking

both nostrils; finally exhale through your right nostril for four seconds. Now do the whole exercise the other way round – inhaling through your right nostril, blocking both nostrils and holding your breath, then releasing and exhaling through your left nostril. This completes one round. I suggest you do six rounds then increase if you would like to.

3 For a more advanced version of the above exercise, add a visualization to increase the prana that is absorbed. Inhale through your left nostril for a count of four, then close both nostrils and retain the breath for a count of four. Then breathe out through your right nostril for a count of six. To complete the round, breathe in through your right nostril for a count of four, block your nostrils and hold the breath for a count of four, then breathe out slowly through your left nostril for a count of six. Use the Chin Lock when you are holding your breath. Do this exercise only if you can do so without straining. As you are holding your breath, imagine that you are sending a current of prana down your spine, through your chakras into your Root Chakra. Remember to keep your breath slow and smooth.

4 Breathe in through both nostrils for a count of two. Hold for a count of four using the Chin Lock, then breathe out for a count of four, releasing the Chin Lock. As you do this, imagine you are absorbing prana as pure energy into your whole body. You might like to think of this as a colour. By using your mind in this way, you are increasing the absorption and circulation of prana. When you use the Chin Lock while you are holding your breath, close your eyes and think about the energy you are storing in your solar plexus. As you breathe out imagine that the current of prana is spreading from your Solar Plexus Chakra to the rest of your body: to every organ, muscle, cell and nerve. Pay special attention to sending prana to your head and think about how it is invigorating and stimulating you. If you have any area you wish to heal, you can send the prana there. Repeat this several times. Really concentrate on this exercise, thinking only of your breath and prana.

5 The first four exercises involve holding the breath after the *inhalation*. In this one you retain the breath after your *exhalation*,

using a breathing pattern called the Square, because of its 4:4:4:4 pattern. Breathe in for a count of four, hold your breath for a count of four, breathe out for four and then hold your breath for another count of four before you start the round again. You can vary this pattern if you like – for example, you can use 6:6:6:6. In addition, you could use the Chin Lock after the inhalation, and the Abdomen and Root Lock when you are holding your breath after the exhalation. You could also try using this square rhythm when you are out walking, using your steps to count. The rhythm here is most important as it prepares you for withdrawing the senses, ready for meditation. Practise a few rounds to start with and increase up to 30.

6 This exercise helps to dispel toxins from the skin by generating heat in the body – you may find that it makes you perspire! Exhale, then inhale slowly for a count of four. Hold your breath for four. Then inhale again for a count of four. Hold the breath again for a count of four, then inhale and hold for another count of four. Exhale very slowly. Do two more rounds of this, then relax.

7 Lie on your back on the floor, or on your bed. Close your eyes and visualize a ball of white healing light above the crown of your head. Use the rhythm 8:4:8:4. As you inhale for a count of eight, feel light coming up through the soles of your feet, passing through your chakras and revitalizing your body, until it meets a ball of white light at the Crown Chakra. Hold your breath for four, then exhale and move the light from the top of your head back down to your feet. Hold your breath. When you start the next round of breathing, use the rhythm to slowly circle the light around your body, from your feet to your head and back again, so that you are surrounded in an egg of white, healing light. This exercise can make you feel really calm, yet at the same time, energized and strong.

The last few exercises are used as a preparation for meditation. If you spend a few months practising pranayama, you will become much calmer and find your concentration improves. In Chapter 9 we will look at meditation in more detail.

5

The Postures – Getting Started

In the next four chapters I shall be covering all the postures in yoga that will help *you* to beat fatigue.

BASIC GUIDELINES

- It is very important to remember that yoga is non-competitive, so work at your own pace without pushing or straining. Be comfortable and relax into the postures.
- Always start with a relaxation posture. Then do some short warm-up stretches. Relax between each posture. And always finish with a relaxation posture such as the Pose of Complete Rest. If you want to beat fatigue there are three important things to learn – relaxation, relaxation and more relaxation! This is not the same as stretching out in front of the TV, but a conscious letting go of muscle tension. I put a lot of emphasis on relaxation as it is something we don't do often enough, and as I explained in Chapter 1 when I talked about stress, tension is a major cause of fatigue. So don't feel guilty – relaxation postures are as important as 'active' postures in yoga. And anyway, yoga is about being, not doing!
- Try to think of each posture as an exercise in meditation. By this I mean that you should become completely involved and concentrate only on the posture so that your mind doesn't

wander. Think about the flow of energy as you breathe. Above all, *enjoy* your yoga practice – think of it as your treat, your time, not just something else on a long list of things that you have to do.

- Breathe through your nose as you work. Remember to breathe normally when you hold a posture. In yoga you work in rhythm with your breath. I'll explain this as we go along, but as a rough rule of thumb, you breathe in when you lift a limb, and out when you lower it.
- Always come out of a posture very carefully, not suddenly or jerkily.
- It is beneficial to repeat a posture two or three times, and to hold it for as long as you feel is right.
- You must check with your doctor first if you have any health problems, including the following: heart trouble, high blood pressure, eye problems such as glaucoma, ear trouble or back problems. (Yoga can help with some back problems, but you need to check with your physiotherapist, chiropractor or osteopath about which exercises are relevant for you – some postures could make your condition worse.) If you are pregnant and haven't done yoga before it's *very* important that you consult a yoga teacher, because some of the postures in this book should not be practised during pregnancy.
- Do not eat for at least two hours before doing any yoga postures. This is because digestion uses up energy. Empty your bladder first. Wear loose, comfortable clothing such as leggings or tracksuit bottoms with a T-shirt or fleece. Ideally you should work in bare feet as you are liable to slip when doing some of the standing postures. If your feet get cold you can wear socks with rubber grips. You may like to use a blanket for relaxation. Make sure you have enough space to work. Switch off the phone so that you won't be disturbed.
- Do not do the inverted postures if you are menstruating or if you have high blood pressure.
- Always, always balance your postures. If you work on your right side, such as in the Triangle, you must work on your left

side too. You must always counterpose – for example, if you do some backward bends, you then need to do some forward bends. As you do more yoga, your body will know when to counterpose; it will start to feel its natural balance so that you will *know* you need to bend forward after you have been bending backwards.

- Try to practise for a minimum of 20 minutes a day. A full yoga session usually lasts 90 minutes. At home, if you can do one hour once a day, that is brilliant. You will see results faster. However, 20 minutes is better than no minutes, and twice a week is better than not at all. Aim to get into a regular routine, perhaps setting your alarm clock earlier and doing your yoga practice first thing in the morning.
- If you have Chronic Fatigue Syndrome, start very slowly and listen to your body all the time. No one else can tell you what your limit is – only you know that. On some days you will be able to do more than on others. The golden rule is never do too much – always do less than you think you can. I suggest that you start off with just a few warm-up stretches for a month, then add one posture a week, depending on how well you are. Progress very slowly and don't hold the postures for too long. You should avoid the standing postures until you feel strong enough to do them. People with CFS tend to be perfectionists – they want to be the best. Think of your yoga practice as learning that you don't need to think like this – your best is what you can manage, and no more.

In this book, as you will have realized, I emphasize prana and pranayama (universal energy, and control of this through breathing). *All* yoga postures are designed to direct prana or vital energy to different parts of the body, and each pose works on one or more of your energy centres or chakras. However, in order to maximize the use of prana, I would like you to approach these postures in a slightly different way. As you do your yoga poses in rhythm with your breathing, I want you to think about and visualize the energy running through your system.

When you do this you will see that visualization and proper

breath control helps the flow of energy in your body. There is scientific evidence that visualizing, or thinking about, a posture increases its effect. Psychologists at Manchester Metropolitan University in the UK have discovered that those who think about doing an exercise can improve their muscle groups by up to an additional 16 per cent, providing they imagine the feeling of the response they would get if they were actually doing the exercise. This is because most of the areas in the brain related to physical movement don't know the difference between doing a task and imagining it! I'm not suggesting that you shouldn't actually do the postures, but I am making the point that if you visualize your yoga poses as you work on them you will have a powerful way of encouraging prana.

Finally, a reminder: doing these yoga postures will help your whole system and lead to better health and energy. You will breathe properly and your circulation, organs, muscles, skeleton, ligaments, joints, spine, digestion, endocrine and nervous system will all be helped. These postures will also help to purify your body by removing toxins, and will make your mind strong as you develop stability and concentration. Yoga will help to bring your body, mind and spirit into harmony – and, best of all, it really will beat fatigue!

WORKING OUT A DAILY ROUTINE

It's very simple. In the next four chapters you will find postures listed under the following headings: Relaxation Postures, Warm-up Exercises, Lying Down Poses, Sitting Postures, Backward Bends, Standing Postures, Twists, and Inverted Postures. Forward bends are included in the Sitting and Standing sections. All you have to do is choose one or two postures from each category to make up your own daily routine. Those marked with one star (*) are easier than those marked with two, so should be practised first before you move on. Try to vary the postures so that you don't do the same ones each time. As you feel stronger you can add more postures from each category. Remember to start and finish a session with relaxation, and to do some warm-up stretches before the poses. As I mentioned, you always need to counter a forward- or backward-bending posture with one that takes you in the opposite direction. If you don't want to make up your own routine, I've included three daily sequences that you can use.

If you are new to yoga or have Chronic Fatigue Syndrome, start with the postures with one star. Only when you feel strong enough should you move on to the two-star postures. In yoga, the more advanced you become, the longer you will be able to hold a posture, so at the beginning, hold the posture just for a few seconds and build up your tolerance slowly. As a very rough guide, you will find that backward bends are energizing and forward bends are calming.

Before you start you may find it easier to record the exercise instructions slowly onto a audio tape so that you can carry out the poses without having to look at the book all the time. Or you might like to ask a friend to read them out to you.

Relaxation Postures*

The Pose of Complete Rest
This posture is also known as The Corpse, the literal translation from the Sanskrit. It is so called because when performed properly both your body and mind should be completely still. We already covered this posture in Chapter 2, but as it is so important I would like to go over it once again. It is said that 20 minutes of relaxation is equivalent to five hours of sleep, so this really is an invaluable posture to practise.

Lie down with your eyes closed. Cover yourself with a blanket if you are cold. Try to relax as much as possible. Let your legs flop apart and rotate slightly outwards. Your palms should be facing upwards, but only if this is comfortable. Some people like to put their hands on their abdomen instead. Now go through each body part, first tensing then relaxing it. Start with your feet and progress up to your legs, hands, arms, neck, shoulders, back, abdomen area, torso, jaws, face, forehead, and the back of your head. Pay particular attention to your shoulders, neck, jaws and abdomen, the areas where most tension is stored. In fact you might like to think of your abdominal area as the hub of a wheel, from where relaxation spreads to all the other parts. You can do this by imagining a soothing, yellow, warm colour expanding outwards from this area, sending relaxing waves to the rest of your body. Really concentrate on each part as you go through the pose, and try not to let your mind wander. Let your breath flow naturally. As you relax, your breathing should become deeper and slower. Feel yourself sinking into your support. Let all tension flow away. Try and hold onto this feeling of being relaxed and carry it with you throughout the day, so that if you become tense, you can consciously relax again.

Quick Tension Reliever
This is an excellent way to relax quickly if you haven't the time to go through the full relaxation sequence.

Lie on the floor. Breathe in and lift your head, legs and arms slightly up from the floor – no more than a few inches. Now, holding your breath, tighten everything as much as possible. Screw up your face, make fists with your hands, clench your buttocks and really grip everything as firmly as you can. Then breathe out with a big sigh – 'haaa' – and let everything flop back onto the floor. Repeat twice more.

Pigeon Hole Visualization
This is another relaxation that is excellent to use at the beginning of a yoga class or meditation practice, when your head may be buzzing from the outside world and all the things you have to do. It is also very good as an aid to concentration.

First, relax as much as you physically can. Close your eyes.

Now, think of all your problems and all the things you have to do. Examine everything that is cluttering up your mind. Imagine that in front of you is a large wooden pigeon-hole unit, like those that hold letters and keys behind the reception desk in a hotel. Now imagine all your problems and responsibilities flying into the pigeon holes. As they do so, a shutter comes down and, for now, your troubles have been put aside and you don't need to think about them. Your mind is clear. If you want you can open just one shutter to concentrate on any task you are doing. (For example, if you are in the car, open the shutter called 'driving' so that you concentrate on that one task and nothing else.) For now, you need to open the shutter called 'yoga postures'. Remind yourself that this is your time to practise yoga and that you can attend to other needs when you finish. For the duration of your session there is nothing to be done, solved or thought about that can't wait until the end of your yoga practice. Your mental pigeon hole has taken away all your thoughts and problems for now.

After your yoga session you can carry on using this mental image so that throughout the day you have just one shutter open related to every task you do. In this way you can focus on what you are doing without worrying about anything else.

The Windmill
This isn't strictly a relaxation posture, but I've included it here because it is very soothing and excellent for breath control.

Stand upright, keeping your shoulders relaxed, and let your arms hang by your side. Now, on an in-breath, swing your arms together towards your abdomen, then lift them up over your head. On an out-breath, circle your arms outwards and down to your sides. Repeat up to five times. Do this very slowly and aim to make big, circling, sweeping movements with your arms. You can do this sitting down if you prefer. Now change direction so that you are circling your arms the other way.

This exercise pumps air and prana into your body and so is also very energizing.

The Pose of a Child
This is an excellent pose to do between postures. If you have problems relaxing on your back, you may like to try this instead.

> Kneel, keeping your hips on your heels. Now stretch forwards and take your forehead down onto the floor. If you like, or if you have high blood pressure, you can rest your head on blocks or a book. Take your arms to the side of your body, with your palms turned up, and relax.

This posture, with your head slightly lower than your heart, helps with blood flow to the brain so that your whole system is energized. As it is a forward bend, this posture can be used to conter a backward bend.

Figure 5   The Pose of a Child

Warm-up Exercises

Basic Stretching
You must always start your yoga practice with a few warm-up stretches so that you don't damage any of your muscles. You can do your stretches lying down or standing up, whichever you prefer.

Lying Down Stretch
Lie down with your eyes closed. Now, on an in-breath, slowly stretch your arms up over your head, stretching your hands away from your shoulders as much as you can. At the same time, stretch out your legs and point your toes. Pull your feet away from your hips. Hold for a few seconds. On an out-breath, sigh 'haaa' and bring your arms back down to your sides and relax everything. Hold for a few seconds, then repeat the stretch twice more.

Incidentally, you sigh 'haaa' because it helps with the expulsion of old, stale air, and the intake of oxygen on the next breath.

Standing Stretches
With your feet just a few inches apart, lift your arms over your head and link your hands together, stretching up towards the ceiling. Keep your hips straight and tilt the upper part of your body over to the right and stretch out. Come back to the centre and stretch up further. Now bend the upper half of your body slightly to the left and stretch. Then come back to the centre. Breathe normally as you do this. Now bend your trunk down and swing your arms towards your feet. If you can touch your toes do so, but only if you can do this without straining. Otherwise, bend your knees slightly so you can reach down. To finish, come up slowly and put your hands on the back of your hips. Slowly lean back from your pelvis, then your waist,

Figure 6   Standing Stretches

your shoulders and finally your head – but don't take it too far.

Neck Roll

We all carry a lot of tension in our neck and shoulders – often without realizing – and this can add to the picture of fatigue. As well as using this exercise for your yoga session, you may like to try it during the day if you feel tension building up. It is particularly good if you work sitting down – such as at a computer or in an office – or if you do a lot of driving.

Find a position that feels comfortable – sitting in a chair, kneeling, or sitting cross-legged. Keep upright, but relaxed. Think about your spine. Is there any tension there? Let go of any tightness without slumping. Think about how your head is positioned on your shoulders. Your head should not be hanging too far forward or straining too far back. Put your fingers on the back of your neck and work out how to hold your head in a way which causes the least tension in your neck. Your head should pivot freely on your atlas joint – where the skull meets the spine – and there should be no compression there. Think of a string coming out of the top of your head, lifting it up towards the ceiling.

Figure 7   Neck Roll

On an out-breath bring your chin slowly down towards
your chest in time with your breath. On an in-breath return
it to the centre. On an out-breath roll your head slightly
back, keeping your jaw closed. Don't take it too far back.
Breathe in and come back to the centre. Repeat this
movement three times. Now breathe in, and on the out-
breath slowly roll your right ear towards your right
shoulder. Breathe in again, and on the next two out-breaths
see if you can take your ear a little further towards your
shoulder. Pause, then on an in-breath bring your head back
to the centre. On an out-breath roll your left ear towards
your left shoulder. Again, see if you can slowly take your
ear a little further towards your shoulder on the next two
out-breaths. On an in-breath bring your head back to the
centre. Repeat this three times. Finally, still sitting upright
and making sure you are not slumping, slowly look over
your right shoulder on an out-breath. Return your head to
the centre, then on the next out-breath gently take your

head a little further to the right. Take your head back to the centre then repeat again. On the third out-breath you should be able to take your head even further round to the right, but don't force it. Repeat on your left side, making sure that your trunk is facing forward and pressing down on the base of the spine to improve the flexibility in your neck.

Shoulder Shrug and Roll

Sit or kneel as in the Neck Roll. Now shrug your shoulders by putting them up towards your ears, then letting them flop down. Do this several times. Each time, as they relax down, they should come further away from your ears. Now gently roll your shoulders in big circles, allowing your arms to flop as you do so. Do this several times, then circle your shoulders the other way. You can bend your arms and put your hands on your shoulders if you prefer. Keep the movements slow, in time with your breathing,

Joint Exercises

The expression 'use it or lose it' is very apposite in relation to joints. These exercises will help to keep your joints supple and

Figure 8   Shoulder Roll

mobile so that if you practise them regularly, you shouldn't suffer from stiffness as you get older.

Elbows and Shoulders

Sit in a comfortable position. Now slowly circle your wrists about five times, then change direction. Next, hold your arms out at shoulder level in a L shape, with your elbows bent and your forearms pointing upwards. Push your hands back. Now keep the upper part of your arm still as you bend your lower or forearms slowly until your hands point downwards. Your arms should still be in an L shape. Push the palms of your hands back. Look at your upper arms to make sure that they haven't dropped.

You will probably hear lots of creaks from your elbows and shoulders, which is a good sign! The tricky thing here is to keep your upper arms as still as possible, otherwise you are not mobilizing your elbows enough.

Figure 9   Joint Exercise

Ankles
Sit on a chair and cross one leg over the other. Stretch your toes forward and back to get some movement in them. Now try and separate your toes, then give them a good wriggle. Next, stretch your heels forward and pull your toes back. Finally, circle your ankle slowly about five times one way, then five times the other way. Change legs.

Knees
Still sitting on your chair, stretch your right leg out in a straight line and flex and point your toes. Now bend your leg, straighten it, bend it and straighten it again. This helps to mobilize the knee. Change over and do the same with the left leg.

Fingers
To mobilize your finger joints, make fists, then straighten your fingers. Repeat several times. Now wriggle your fingers as if you were playing the piano, or typing quite fast. Finally, give your fingers a good shake.

Pelvic Lift
This is a good exercise for mobilizing the pelvis, and one that will help you later when you are learning the Mountain Pose, which is about good posture. It is also beneficial for the pelvic floor muscles and the waist, and will help you in forward stretching postures.

Lie on the floor on your back with your legs bent at the knees, hip-width apart, with your ankles under your knees. Relax, then on an in-breath, start to press your waist into the floor. As you do so, your hips and pelvic area will start to rise slightly so you are titling your pelvis back; your hips should still be on the floor. Hold for a few seconds, keeping the waist area tight. Now on an out-breath, slowly roll the hips down and relax.

When you have finished this pelvic movement, bring your knees to your chest and have a gentle rock from side to side. Then, with one hand on each knee and the knees together, slowly circle your knees first one way then the other. This gives a good massage to the back of the spine.

The above exercises are all excellent ways of easing and stretching before you start your full yoga session. In the next chapter we will be looking at yoga postures that are specifically designed to give you more energy and vitality.

6

Postures to Energize and Revitalize

Now that you have relaxed, stretched and warmed up, you are ready to start practising the poses.

Lying Down Postures

Head to Knee Pose*
This is a gentle forward stretch, so you need to counter this movement with a backward bend. This pose helps to tone the bowel and to prevent constipation, wind and irritable bowel syndrome.

Lie on your back with your legs out straight. Now bend your right leg and bring it towards your chest, hugging it with your right arm so it is in the crook of your elbow with your arm over your knee. Keep everything relaxed on your left side. Next, on an in-breath, and taking special care if you have neck or shoulder problems, lift your head up towards your knee. Hold for a few seconds, breathing normally. On an out-breath lower your head, then breathe in. On another out-breath lower your knee and stretch your leg out straight. Repeat three times then do the same on your left side.

Figure 10   Head to Knee Pose

Leg Raises*

Lie down on the floor on your back with your legs stretched out. On an in-breath, slowly lift your right leg towards the ceiling. Keep your leg as straight as possible and bring it as near as you can towards your head without straining. If you find this is too much, you can bend your left leg, which will make the pose easier. If on the other hand you are quite supple, you can hold onto your lower leg with your hands and gently bring your leg further towards your head to increase the stretch. Flex your foot towards the ceiling so that your heel is stretching up, which will also increase the stretch. Breathe out. Now, breathing in and holding onto your leg, gently lift your head up towards your leg and stretch your leg further towards your head. If you have any

Figure 11   Leg Raises

neck or shoulder problems, do this last part carefully. On an out-breath, lower your head, breathe in, then on the next out-breath slowly lower your leg. Do twice more, then repeat on your left side.

The Fish*
The Fish is a backward-bend movement so is therefore a very useful counter posture for forward bends such as the Head to Knee Pose. It is also used as a counterpose to the Shoulder Stand and the Half Shoulder Stand, which I will be explaining later. The Fish, is an excellent posture for increasing vital energy to the Heart Chakra because it opens the chest fully. It is also a good posture for breathing problems such as asthma and can help to correct hunched or rounded shoulders.

Sit upright with your legs outstretched and lean back on your elbows and forearms so that they are supporting you. Pull in the back of your pelvis. Look up at the wall and curve the back of your waist. Look higher up the wall to curve your spine in towards your shoulder blades. Finally, ease your elbows a little further forward towards your hips until you can gently bring the crown of your head to rest lightly on the floor, or on blocks or books. The pressure on your head *must* be light – your arms should be taking most of your weight.

To work on this posture from the floor when you are more experienced, you can try this:

Lie on the floor with your feet together and your arms by your side. Now, on an in-breath, press slightly on your

Figure 12   The Fish

forearms, arch your back and slide onto the back of your head. Raise your chest area as high as you can. Keep your legs as relaxed as possible. Breathe deeply, keeping your waist area held in. To make the posture stronger, push your elbows into the floor to help open the chest even more. Remember, you should not be putting too much pressure on your head. Hold for 30 seconds, increasing this time only when you feel able to do so without straining. Breathe out to come out of the posture.

The Bridge*
This back bend resembles the span of a bridge. It is excellent for tightening the abdominal area, strengthening the back and keeping the spine flexible.

Lie flat with your knees bent and your arms by your side, palms face down. Your feet should be about hip-width apart. Keeping your feet on the floor, with your ankles under your knees, breathe out and slowly lift up your hips and move onto your shoulders so that you form an arch. Keep your neck and head on the floor. Tighten behind your knees, thighs, buttocks and lower back. Use your arms to support you by keeping them pushed down under your 'bridge', and press down hard with your feet. Lift your hips as high as you can. If you want to increase the lift, you can hold under your waist with your hands and push up, which will take you further onto your shoulders. Remember to breathe normally and hold the pose for a few

Figure 13   The Bridge

seconds. Come out of the posture on an in-breath, rolling your back down very slowly, vertebra by vertebra, onto the floor. Repeat twice more.

Sitting postures

Sitting Forward Stretch*
This is a forward bend, so will need to be couterposed with a backward bend.

> Sit on the floor with your legs outstretched. Try and sit upright but without any tension in your back – in other words, don't slump. Keep your heels together and your toes flexed. Now inhale, raise your arms up over your head and, bending back slightly, look up at your hands. Exhale and slowly bend forward from the hips – not the waist – so that your breastbone is in line with your legs. Just bend a little way and then, on an in-breath, raise your arms up over your head again and stretch up. Now, bending from the hips again on an out-breath, fold forwards a little further. Come up again on an in-breath, stretch your arms up further towards the ceiling then fold your arms and trunk down as far as you can on the next out-breath, keeping your spine in a straight line. If you are very flexible, you will be able to rest your trunk on your thighs and your arms on your calves, or even the floor. Breathe normally and relax. If you can't stretch this far forwards, don't worry – just go as far as you can. You are aiming to

Figure 14   Sitting Forward Stretch

keep your trunk straight whilst stretching forward, so don't curve your spine in order to get further. Hold for a few seconds, relaxing and breathing deeply; this helps to generate energy in your Solar Plexus Chakra. Come out of the posture slowly on an in-breath.

This forward bend benefits your internal organs and the nervous system. Whilst performing this posture, remember the saying that applies to all yoga: 'Don't sprain – if pain, no gain!'

The Head of a Cow – also known as Hand Clasp*

Like the Fish, this posture is very good for opening out the chest area and bringing vital energy to the Heart Chakra. It is also good for toning the upper part of the arm, or 'batwing' arms. It benefits the shoulders and gives an excellent diagonal stretch to your back.

Kneel, so that you are sitting upright on the back of your heels. Now take your left arm up behind your back and

Figure 15   The Head of a Cow

bend it so that your hand is between your shoulder blades, pointing up your back as far as it can reach. Take your right hand down over your right shoulder so that the hands meet and you can grip your fingers together. If you can't reach this far, don't worry – use a belt, handkerchief or sock between your two hands. Pull up and down on your hands to increase the diagonal stretch in your back. Hold for about ten breaths. Now repeat on the other side.

Most people can reach further on one side than the other. This is because it is usually more difficult to twist your dominant arm (ie the right if you are right handed) into the upward position.

The Lion*
This pose is called the Lion because that is what you'll look like – you make a really fierce face! It is very beneficial if you are suffering from a sore throat or feel you are about to get a cold. It also stimulates blood and vital energy to your face, helping to

Figure 16   The Lion

conteract feelings of lethargy. It will actually help to make you a better colour if you are usually very pale. It's not difficult to do – and is particularly good if you have CFS.

Kneel, resting upright on the backs of your heels. Place the palms of your hands on your knees, with your fingers splayed, and take a deep breath in through your nose. Now lean forward slightly and breathe out forcefully through your mouth, making a 'haaa' sound. As you do so, stretch your tongue out and down, stretch out your fingers, and look up to the point between your eyebrows. Hold the pose for a few seconds then close your mouth and breathe normally. Repeat twice more.

The Boat**

This posture is very good for firming your abdominal muscles and your back, which in turn will help to support your spine.

Sit upright on the floor, with your legs straight in front of you. Now breathe out, and on the next in-breath, take your legs up into the air. Your feet should be slightly higher than your eye level. You should be resting on the base of your spine so that your body forms a V shape. Stretch your arms out in front of you, outside your legs. Hold the posture for

Figure 17   The Boat

a few seconds – you should feel your abdominal muscles working. Breathe deeply. To increase prana or vitality, make rowing motions with your arms. This helps to pump energy into your body, particularly your Solar Plexus Chakra, which is your energy or sun centre. To come out of the position, reverse the movements on an out-breath. Repeat twice more.

The Canoe**
You need firm abdominal muscles for this next pose, so don't try it unless you have been practising yoga regularly for a few months.

Lie on your back with your feet together. Stretch your arms along the floor over your head, with your palms together. Breathe in and raise your head, arms, legs and shoulders about 15 inches from the floor. Hold for about five seconds then breathe out as you come down very slowly. Repeat twice more if you wish.

Make sure you relax for a few minutes after this posture – you will need to!

Figure 18   The Canoe

The Butterfly*
The Butterfly is a good posture to practise in preparation for the Lotus position. I won't be covering the Lotus position in this book, but if you join a yoga class, you will be taught the Half Lotus and, when you are very advanced, the Full Lotus. (In the

Figure 19   The Butterfly

Half Lotus you sit cross-legged with one foot tucked up by the opposite thigh). Sitting upright helps prana to flow along the spine, and this posture helps ankles, knees and hips to become more flexible.

Sit upright on your sitting bones – ie not slumping on the base of your spine but sitting up on your buttocks. Clasp your feet together. Now gently bounce your knees up and down. You are aiming to get your knees as near to the floor as you can, and it will help if you visualize your knees going further as you practise this. Do this movement for about two minutes, then put a hand on each knee and gently press them down.

Backward Bends

As I mentioned in Chapter 5, backward bends are very energizing; they are also used to counter forward-bend movements such as the Sitting Forward Stretch.

Figure 20   The Sphinx

The Sphinx*
This is one of my favourite postures – there is a very solid feel
to it.

Lie on your front on your abdomen and hips, so that the
upper half of your body is lifted from the floor. Rest on your
forearms making sure that your elbows are directly under
your shoulders. Pull your shoulders back towards your feet
and lift the crown of your head towards the ceiling so that
your breastbone is in a vertical position. Your arms should
form a square shape. Don't allow your shoulders to slump
or tighten. Look straight ahead and hold for a few seconds,
focusing on your lumbar area (the base of your spine).
Breathe normally. Come down slowly on an out-breath,
rest, and then repeat twice.

The Cobra**
When you are confident enough with the Sphinx, you can
progress to this next posture. The Cobra looks simple, but it is
very easy to get wrong. Don't be tempted to push yourself up
with your hands, thus compressing the curve at the back of your
waist. Your upper back should be lengthened – keep in mind the
image of a snake as you practise this.

Lie down with your forehead on the floor, arms by your side
with your palms facing up. Now rest your forearms and
palms on the floor under your shoulders. If you haven't

Figure 21   The Cobra

done this posture before, put your hands wherever is comfortable, which may be in front of your shoulders. As you progress, you can move your hands nearer your chest, or under your shoulders with your fingers facing forwards. On an in-breath slowly start to lift up your trunk. Lift from the hips using your back muscles, rather than pushing up with your hands. As you lift, brush your chin and nose along the floor so that you are leading with your head. Drop your hips and lengthen forward as you lift up the upper part of your body, opening your chest and abdomen. Try and keep your shoulders dropped and soft, not hunched or stiff. Look straight ahead and breathe normally. Hold the posture for a few seconds then reverse the procedure slowly to come down. Relax, and then repeat if you wish.

This is quite a strong backward bend so it should follow a forward bend, or be followed by one.

The Cobra is very beneficial: it can help to alleviate menstrual problems, to stimulate the adrenal glands and the kidneys, and to improve spinal strength and flexibility – and therefore posture. It generates energy in both the Heart and the Root Chakra.

If you have CFS and experience swings of energy or sometimes feel hypermanic, I suggest you stick to the Sphinx and avoid the Cobra.

The Locust

Half Locust*
Lie on your front with your arms to the side with your palms facing upwards. Make fists with your hands. Keep your chin on the floor. Inhale and raise your right leg, keeping the body and leg straight. Exhale and lower your leg. Do the same on your left side. Repeat three times on both sides. Now raise your right leg and keep it up for as long as is comfortable, breathing normally. Exhale and slowly lower the leg. Repeat on the other side, then do twice more on both sides.

Figure 22(a)   Half Locust

Full Locust**
From the same starting position as the Half Locust, make fists with your hands and place your arms under your body, so that your fists are under your hips. Keeping your chin touching the floor, push down with your fists and raise both legs up from the floor. Breathe normally and hold the position for a few seconds, then on an out-breath, slowly lower the legs.

Figure 22(b)   Full Locust

The Locust strengthens the abdominal muscles, aids digestion and gastric disorders, strengthens the lower back, helps the bladder and prostrate gland, and is also excellent for varicose veins. It is classed as a semi-inverted posture and helps to bring blood to the face.

The Bow***

This posture raises both halves of the body together, combining the effect of both the Locust and the Cobra. Consequently, it is excellent for toning the back muscles, improving the health of the spine, and increasing energy. It also helps the digestive and reproductive systems and gives the internal organs a massage.

> Lie down on your front with your head down. Bend your knees up so that your feet are towards your buttocks. Now reach back with your hands and clasp your ankles. Breathe out. Inhale and raise your head and chest, holding your ankles. Lift your knees, thighs, hips and lower back so that your knees come up from the floor, your heels move away from your buttocks and your toes point up towards the ceiling. You should be resting on your abdomen. Arch backwards and look up or, if this strains your neck, straight ahead. Take three deep breaths to stimulate energy to your Solar Plexus Chakra; you may find you rock slightly as you breathe in and out. Exhale and come down slowly. Repeat twice more, then relax into the Pose of a Child.

Figure 23   The Bow

7

Postures to Aid Relaxation and Increase Stamina

This chapter covers standing postures and twists; some of these poses are quite strong, so practise them only if you already have a certain amount of stamina and flexibility, especially if you suffer from Chronic Fatigue Syndrome.

Standing Postures

The Mountain Pose*
This pose will help you to stand with good posture. It is essentially a standing still posture, but don't be deceived – like the Pose of Complete Rest there is a lot more to it, and you need to be completely involved to do it properly. This posture forms the basis for all the other standing postures, and you should try to apply it whenever you are standing during the day – waiting in a queue, walking, and so on.

Stand up straight with your arms by your sides. Close your eyes. Breathe slowly and relax. Think about your feet and feel your balance so that you are not too far forward over your toes, or too far back over your heels. Keep your legs slightly apart and your knees soft. Now think about your pelvis. If you wear high heels or carry heavy loads, it is very common for your pelvis to be tilted too far forward. In fact it should be slightly back, with your bottom tucked under. Now think about your back. Is it straight, or are you rounding your spine? Try and keep it upright without causing strain. Think of your back stretching up. If you were taught that good posture involves holding your shoulders back and thrusting your chest out, this is incorrect for it causes excessive tension. Instead, think about your shoulders being relaxed and falling away from your ears. Now think about your head. Check that there is no tension in your neck and that your head is balanced as it should be – rising up gently from your spine. Your atlas joint, where your head pivots on your neck, is often a point of stress, but because it is a channel for all the main nerves and arteries to the brain, it needs to be relaxed. Your head and your body should be in a straight line, as if a piece of taut string is running up your back and head to the ceiling. Feel yourself rooted in the earth with your feet, with your

Figure 24   The Mountain Pose

head lifting up to the sky. You should be aware of how your posture feels, but also relaxed – there should be no tension in any part of you. Breathe normally for a minute or two, then lift your arms up over your head, slowly on the in-breath, stretching upwards, then bring them slowly down to your sides on your next out-breath. Repeat five times.

Sideways Bend*

There are four basic movements of the spine: forwards, backwards, sideways and twisting. The sideways movement is important because it opens up each side of the chest and abdomen. It is also very good for improving the flexibility of the spine. The Sideways Bend is a very good preparation for the classic yoga pose, the Triangle, which we will be doing next.

Stand with your feet apart, toes forward, inhale, and raise

Figure 25   Sideways Bend

your arms level with your shoulders. Exhale slowly and lower your right arm, sliding it down your leg towards your calf if you can. Keep your pelvis facing forward. Raise your left arm above your head with the palm inward, so the arm is near your ear. Bend to the right to take your right arm further down your leg. Hold for a few seconds, breathing normally, then inhale to come out of the posture. Repeat on the left side.

The Triangle*
The Triangle is another pose that looks deceptively simple, but is difficult to get right. The temptation is to aim for the floor or your ankle with your hand, allowing the opposite hip and shoulder to tilt forwards. If you do this, you won't benefit from the sideways stretch. I would recommend that you practise this keeping your back against a wall, so that you

Figure 26   The Triangle

know your hips and shoulders are square on and facing forwards.

Stand with your feet wider than hip-width apart (about 1 metre (3 feet)) with your right foot turned out and your left foot turned in just a little. Check that your right heel is in line with the centre of your left foot. Inhale, and then raise your arms parallel to the floor. Turn the palm of your right hand up and push out to the right, as if you were trying to push the wall away. On your next out-breath, lower your right hand to your thigh and slide it as far down your leg as you can, without allowing the left hip or shoulder to swivel forwards. Don't worry if you can't get your hand very far down your leg. Take your left arm up to the ceiling and look up at your thumb. Remember to keep your left hip well back. Hold, breathing normally for as long as it feels comfortable. Inhale, bring your arms up, then exhale and lower your arms to your sides. Repeat on your left side, making sure that you change your feet position accordingly.

Standing Forward Stretch*
We've already done the Sitting Forward Stretch and now you are going to learn the Forward Stretch from a standing position. This is very useful if you want to counterpose a back bend – and it gives great flexibility to the spine and tones the abdominal muscles. It also helps increase blood flow to the brain, which will give you a huge boost of energy.

Stand in the Mountain pose described at the beginning of this chapter. On an out-breath, lift your arms up over your head, as high as you can. On your next out-breath bend slowly forward from the hips – not the waist – and stretch out your arms in front of you so that they are horizontal with the floor. You can help this movement by pushing your hips and buttocks back to stretch your spine. This will help you to go further forward and stop you curving your

Figure 27 Standing Forward Stretch

back. Now, folding from the hips, come down as far as possible, keeping your back straight. Hold on to your calves with your hands. If you are very flexible you will be able to reach your feet, or even the floor. Keep your weight forward to keep your legs vertical, and make sure your neck and shoulders are relaxed. Don't bend your knees – reach only as far as you can without straining. Hold the pose for about ten breaths – and each time you breathe out, imagine your head coming nearer to the ground and your chest coming nearer to your legs. On an in-breath come up by putting your hands on your hips and slowly uncurling.

The Woodchopper*

This movement is very good for dispelling anger or tension, which both cause fatigue. It really does work – if something is bothering you or making you really cross, try doing this ten times and you will be amazed how your negative emotions disperse!

Stand in the Mountain pose with your feet wide apart. Bend forward slightly and clasp your hands together in front of you, as if you were grabbing an imaginary axe. Now raise your hands above your head on an in-breath. On the next out-breath rigorously swing your axe down towards your feet, taking your arms through your legs and saying 'haaaa' as loudly as you can. Repeat five to ten times.

When you have finished, you may like to relax in the Pendulum pose, which is excellent for releasing tension in the shoulders – another cause of fatigue.

The Pendulum*

Hang forward like a rag doll so that your fingertips are just above the floor. Using your trunk and shoulders, swing you arms from left to right in a rhythmic swinging motion. Then stop swinging and let your arms slow down, making no attempt to control their movement. Wait until they have stopped and then swing them again.

The Tree*

The Tree posture is very good for balance and for concentration, which is a good discipline to develop before you learn to meditate. It is helpful to visualize that you are a tree, with your feet rooted in the ground and your arms like branches reaching to the sky. This then benefits all your chakras.

To get your balance, you need to be relaxed and standing in the Mountain pose. From this starting position you should then be able to stand on one leg without falling over! It will help you to balance if you fix your gaze on something in front of you and concentrate on that point without allowing your attention to wander.

From the Mountain pose shift your weight slightly onto your left leg. Now take your right leg up and tuck it into your left thigh. Tuck your heel into your groin – it's best not to wear socks as the foot tends to slip down. At first you may need to hold your foot in position with your hand, but

Figure 28   The Tree

try and take your hand away if you can. Try to keep your right knee pointing out to the side and don't allow it to come forward. It may help your balance if you place your left hand on your left hip so that your elbow is out to the side, or if you hold your arms out vertically as if you were walking a tightrope. When you feel confident, on an in-breath take you hands in the prayer position and hold them on your chest. Hold for up to ten breaths, breathing normally, then on another in-breath take your arms up over your head with your fingertips touching. Remember to concentrate on looking straight ahead. Hold this position for ten breaths. As you get more confident you can extend the time you hold your Tree posture. Repeat on the other side.

The Eagle**

The Eagle, a more advanced form of the Tree posture, twists and squeezes the spine, increasing circulation to the limbs. It is very good for varicose veins and will help to strengthen your leg muscles.

Stand in the Mountain pose. Slightly bend your left leg. Now wrap your right leg around your left leg from the front. Lean forward slightly and bend your arms so that your palms are facing upwards. Entwine your right arm around the outside of your left arm and hold the palms together. Squeeze your arms and legs together. Now, if you can, rest your elbow on your thigh, with your chin resting on the back of your hand. If you can't do this, just bend down as low as you can. Hold the pose for a few seconds, remembering to breathe, then untwine. Now repeat on the other side.

Figure 29   The Eagle

The Dancer**

Stand in the Mountain pose. Take your weight over on to your left leg, spreading your toes. Bend your right knee and lift your foot back towards your buttocks. Extend your right arm back and hold your ankle. Tuck your tailbone under and draw the shoulder blades together. Breathe in, raising your left arm up to the ceiling close to your left ear, feeling your spine lengthen and keeping both hips level. Breathe out, pivot forward on your hip joints and begin to lean forward slowly, extending the right leg and arm behind and lowering the outstretched left arm to just above shoulder level. Keep looking forward. To increase the stretch, raise your right leg higher on each out-breath. Hold this pose for as long as your balance and breath are steady. To come out of the pose, inhale then lower your right leg, still holding the ankle. On the next out-breath lower your left arm, release your foot and

Figure 30   The Dancer

stand back in the Mountain pose to centre yourself. Repeat on the other side.

Twists

In Chapter 5 I said that for your yoga session you should pick at least one posture from each section. I am including only two basic twists here – a supine and a sitting twist – but it is very important to include a twist in each session as it will both stimulate your spinal nerves and mobilize and increase flexibility in the spine. (You will remember the emphasis I put on spinal mobility and posture and their contribution to your energy levels.) It is also said that twisting the spine stimulates circulation, stimulates the internal organs, breaks down fatty tissue, eliminates toxins – and generally increases prana. So there are many reasons to incorporate twists into your daily routine!

Crocodile Twist*
Lie down on your back, with your arms out at shoulder level. Keep your knees together and bend them so that the soles of your feet are under your knees. Now roll over slowly on an out-breath so that your knees are pointing to the right and your left hip is lifted. Look over your left shoulder to your hand. On an in-breath, return your legs and head to the centre, then on the next out-breath lift your right hip and roll your knees to the left and your head to the right. Breathe in and come back to the centre. Your knees and head should move simultaneously. Keep this a continuous, smooth and slow movement in time with your breath until you have done about five twists to each side.

Always move slowly and smoothly – don't jerk and always remember to practise on both sides. Remember to breathe out as you turn to the side, and in as you come back to the centre. With all the lying down twists it is important to keep your shoulders

Figure 31   Crocodile Twist

anchored to the floor while you try to raise your upper hip as far as you can to increase the twist; this gives a diagonal stretch to your back. There are several variations of this movement. You can include just one – or do them all.

Variations

1 Do the Crocodile Twist as before, but keep your feet and knees wider than hip-width apart. This gives an excellent stretch to the thighs and is very good for the circulation and for eliminating toxins.

2 Lie on your back with your arms out parallel at shoulder level. Keeping your legs straight, cross your left ankle over your right. As in the previous sequence, lift your left hip, twist to the right and turn your head the other way to look at your left hand. Roll back to the centre on an in-breath then twist to the left on the next out-breath, taking your head to the right.

3 Put your right ankle on your left knee. Lift your left hip a little so that your right knee can stretch to the floor on your right side. Turn your head to the left and look at

your hand. Now take your right knee over to your left side, allowing the foot to pivot across the knee towards the floor to give it more leverage. Lift the hip and turn your head to look at your right hand. Do this five times on each side.

When you have finished your Crocodile Twists, hug your knees to your chest and have a gentle rock from side to side. As well as being a relaxing movement, this massages the lower back.

Sitting Twist*
Sit on the floor with your legs outstretched. Sit upright on your sitting bones so that you are not slumped. Now bring your right leg over your left leg and place your foot level with the outside of the left knee. Hold your right ankle with your right hand and place your left hand on the floor behind you in line with your spine. Turn your head to look over your left shoulder, gently squeezing your left shoulder blade back against your spine. Work upwards from the base

Figure 32   Sitting Twist

of your spine so that as you make the movement, your spine lengthens and the left side of your abdomen lifts, followed by your ribs and chest. Sit upright as you rotate your body. Breathe normally as you hold the pose, twisting slightly further round on each out-breath. Repeat on the other side.

To increase the stretch – if you are flexible enough – after you have brought the right leg over the left, stretch forwards and bring your left elbow to rest on the outside of your right knee, using your hand to hold the ankle. Now take your right arm behind your back so that it is resting on your waist. Check that your shoulders are back and not too tight. Turn your head and look over your left shoulder and hold the posture for a few minutes, breathing normally from your rib area using your diaphragm. Untwist gradually on an in-breath, then repeat on the other side.

In the next chapter we will be learning inverted postures – which are vital for energy – and looking at a sequence that has been designed especially to beat fatigue.

8

Postures to Beat Fatigue

Inverted Postures

In an inverted posture you are either upside down or your head
is lower than your heart. These poses are incredibly beneficial in
combating fatigue as blood circulation is generally improved
and therefore circulation to the brain is encouraged. I haven't
included the Headstand because it is difficult for beginners and
I think it should be attempted only under supervision, although
it is said to be one of the most important of all yoga postures.
However, the Full Shoulder Stand and Half Shoulder Stand are
just as useful. Both can help remedy a variety of complaints such
as low blood pressure, varicose veins and leg aches. They also
help to eliminate waste matter in the lower bowel. Best of all,
because you have to keep the chin tucked in, the thyroid gland
is invigorated, and this in turn stimulates the production of
various hormones from the endocrine system, including
thyroxine. A lack of thyroxine is associated with poor energy, as
you may remember from Chapter 1. Associated with this chin
position is a new chakra (identified in the 20th century) at
the point between the breast and the neck. It is related to the
immune system, which means that the Shoulder Stand can also
help to regulate your immune function. The chin position used
for this yoga posture also involves the Chin Lock (described in
Chapter 4) to help seal in prana and energize your whole system.

All this makes the Shoulder Stand sound too good to be true – a 'cure all' posture – but it really will help to improve your health and energy if you practise it regularly. If you have high blood pressure, or goitre, heart, lung, eye or ear conditions, please check with your doctor before you try any inverted postures. Don't practise these postures if you are menstruating.

Half Shoulder Stand*

Lie on your back with your arms by your sides and your palms down. Aim to keep your body as relaxed as possible. Breathing in, take your legs and trunk into the air, bringing your hips off the ground. Immediately support your hips with your hands so that your legs and hips are at an angle of about 45 degrees to your trunk. Hold this position, keeping your neck and shoulders relaxed, and breathe normally for about a minute, increasing the time as you feel stronger. Keep your legs and toes relaxed. Remember not to strain – if you feel uncomfortable, come out of the posture. If it's easier, rest your legs on a chair. This isn't cheating – you are still getting

Figure 33   Half Shoulder Stand

the same benefits. To come out of the posture, breathe in, and then on an out-breath slowly roll your hips onto the floor.

Full Shoulder Stand**
Once you have practised and mastered the Half Shoulder Stand, you can move on to the full version of this posture.

Lie on your back with your arms to the side and your palms down. Breathing in, swing your legs and hips from the floor. Lift your feet up to the ceiling until your body is straight, working yourself carefully onto your shoulders. Immediately support your back with your hands, keeping them parallel so that your spine doesn't twist. Keep your elbows as close together as possible. Tuck your chin into your chest. Don't sink into your hands but keep your spine as erect as you can so that you are reaching up towards the ceiling, but without strain. Relax into the posture as much as possible whilst keeping this upright position. Breathe normally. To come out of the posture breathe out and slowly bring your knees

Figure 34   Full Shoulder Stand

towards your chest. Arch your neck to keep your head down and roll your spine and hips down slowly onto the floor. Rest for at least as long as you held the posture.

Because you have stretched your neck vertebrae forwards, you must counter this posture by doing the Fish, the Sphinx or the Cobra.

The Pose of Tranquillity*
This posture is so called because it can help you with relaxation and is very good for insomnia – try it if you can't sleep at night.

Lie on the floor and raise your trunk and legs as described in the Shoulder Stand sequence. Now, on an in-breath, start to lower your legs behind your head – without bending them – until they are at a 45-degree angle to the floor. You should feel a point of balance somewhere between the base of your neck and your shoulder blades. When you feel this balance, bring up your arms and hold your ankles or shins. Hold this position for a minute or two, preferably keeping your eyes closed. Remember to breathe normally. Try and develop a peaceful, floating feeling.

From this pose you can go into the Plough, described next.

Figure 35   The Pose of Tranquillity

The Plough**

This posture has all the benefits of the Shoulder Stand, but it also gives flexibility to the neck and shoulders, nourishes the spine, releases tension and massages the internal organs.

It is best to approach the Plough from the Shoulder Stand or Pose of Tranquillity. From either of these positions, with your hips off the floor and ensuring that you are supporting your back with your hands, keep your legs straight and slowly bring your feet down towards the floor behind your head. This may be difficult at first so just take your legs back as far as they will reach without strain. When you first learn this posture it is best to place a pile of books or blocks behind your head for your feet to rest on. As you get more flexible, you can reduce the pile and work further towards the floor by pushing your hips back with your hands so that you are balanced on your shoulders. You can then take your hands away from your back and lie your arms out vertically on the floor in the opposite direction to your legs. Try and keep your knees straight so that your legs are parallel to the ground, and increase the stretch by tucking your toes under and pushing back with your heels. Hold for as long as is comfortable then come out very slowly on an in-breath, rolling down as you did in the Shoulder Stand.

Figure 36   The Plough

The Cat*

The Cat is not an inverted posture, but is a good pose to do before the Dog Stretch – which is. The Cat pose mimics a cat stretching and is a wonderful posture for easing the spine. It can help all kinds of back problems – including tension in the neck and shoulders – and generally aids spine flexibility and so therefore helps to increase energy.

> Kneel in an all-fours position with your hands directly underneath your shoulders and your thighs vertical and slightly apart. Keep your back relaxed but flat. Your neck should be relaxed, with your head parallel to the floor. Now inhale, look up and hollow your spine so that your abdomen is stretching down towards the floor. Press down on your hands. Remember to do this slowly. Now exhale and slowly arch your spine up towards the ceiling, as high as it will go. Bring your chin in to your chest. Again, hold for a few seconds. Repeat this sequence ten times, breathing in slowly to hollow, then out to arch, and timing this movement of arching and hollowing your spine with your breath. Keep your elbows straight throughout the movement.

If you have been sitting at a desk for a long time, or working at a computer, this is a very good sequence to refresh yourself and stretch the spine. Practise it whenever you can take a five-minute break.

Figure 37   The Cat

The Lying Dog Stretch
This is a lovely relaxation posture to use when you have finished
the Cat stretch.

From your all-fours position, sit back so that your hips are
on your heels, then stretch the front part of your body
forwards, resting your head on the floor. Stretch your arms
out in front of you. Now relax for a few minutes.

Figure 38   The Lying Dog Stretch

The Standing Dog Stretch*
This pose is great for stiffness and is an effective way to stretch
the spinal column, open and release the shoulders, and
stretch the hamstring muscles in the back of the legs. You may
well have short hamstrings if you lead a sedentary life, which
means you will get tired very quickly if you do any walking.
Like the other inverted postures, your head is lower than your
heart in this pose, which increases circulation to the brain and
therefore energy levels.

Start from a 'table' position so that you are kneeling on the
ground with your hands beneath your shoulders and your
thighs vertical – as you were for the Cat. Tuck your toes
under and, on an out-breath, straighten your knees and lift
your hips up towards the ceiling. You should now be in an
inverted V shape. Exaggerate this movement so that your
tailbone is lifting and pointing up to the ceiling to increase
the stretch in your legs. Push with your palms, breathe
evenly and relax your neck and shoulders. Look at your
abdomen. Raise your heels. If you want to increase the lift

Figure 39   The Standing Dog Stretch

further, slowly work your heels to the ground, as if you were pedalling. To increase the stretch even more, you can ease your abdomen towards your thighs, remembering to keep your hips lifted – don't sink down. Hold for as long as you feel comfortable, then come down on an out-breath into the Pose of a Child.

The Rabbit*

The Rabbit, also known as the Hare, has many of the advantages of the other inverted postures, but is much easier and quite gentle – so you may prefer to do this instead. It is the first step towards the Headstand and gets you used to holding your head upside down.

From the Pose of a Child lift your hips up from your heels and roll on to the top of your head. You may like to put a cushion under your head for this. Hold your shins with your hands or, if you prefer, keep your hands on the floor under your shoulders. Hold this position for as long as you feel comfortable, breathing normally. Rest in the Pose of a Child again for a few minutes, then repeat.

Figure 40   The Rabbit

A Simple Sequence to Increase Energy*

My yoga teacher Margo Dixon introduced me to this sequence. It is a lovely set of postures for making you feel revitalized. If you are doing this sequence at home, you can say the words silently to yourself, but articulating these positive words out loud can have a beneficial effect and help to raise your vitality.

1 Stand in the Mountain pose with your arms stretched out horizontal to the floor. Increase the stretch by visualizing that you are pushing the walls away with your hands. Say out loud: 'I am healthy.'
2 Now bend your knees slightly and bend your arms at the elbows with your hands pointing upwards. Say out loud: 'I am strong.'
3 Next, stretch your arms up to the ceiling and come up onto your toes, so that you are reaching up as high as you can. Now say: 'I am full of vitality.'
4 Come down from your toes and wrap your arms around yourself in a hug. Say: 'I am safe.'
5 Finally, come back to the Mountain pose, circle your arms up over your head, and down by your sides as you did in the Windmill posture. As you do this say: 'All is well in my world.'

Figure 41(a)   'I am healthy'

Figure 41(b)   'I am strong'

Figure 41(c)   'I am full of vitality'

Figure 41(d)   'I am safe'

Figure 41(e)   'All is well in my world'

SOME SUGGESTIONS FOR DAILY ROUTINES

In Chapter 5, I suggested that you might like to make up your own daily routines, based on how much time you have, how supple you are and how much stamina you have. Yoga should be tailored to the individual – in other words, chose a routine that suits *you*.

I am going to give you three sets of sequences that you might like to use if you don't want to make your own. Try to vary these so that you do a different one each time you practise.

Day 1
The Pose of Complete Rest
Quick Tension Reliever
Head to Knee Pose
Leg raises
The Cat
Half Shoulder Stand
The Pose of Tranquillity
The Boat or The Canoe
Shoulder and neck exercises
The Head of a Cow
The Sphinx
The Standing Dog Stretch
The Lying Dog Stretch
The Pose of a Child
The Pose of Complete Rest

Day 2
The Pose of Complete Rest
Joint exercises
The Butterfly
Full Shoulder Stand
The Plough
The Fish
Sitting Forward Stretch
The Windmill
Sideways Bend or The Triangle
The Sphinx or The Cobra
The Locust
The Bow
Sitting Twist
The Pose of Complete Rest

Day 3
The Pose of Complete Rest

Crocodile Twist
The Bridge
Full Shoulder Stand
The Plough
The Fish
Standing Forward Stretch
The Mountain Pose
The Tree or The Eagle
The Dancer
The Woodchopper
The Cobra
The Standing Dog Stretch
The Lying Dog Stretch
The Rabbit
The Pose of Complete Rest

Remember to practise your yoga postures regularly and to visualize prana filling your body with energy. You also need to practise yoga breathing on a regular basis if you really want to see a difference in your energy levels. Next we will look at meditation, which will help to increase your stamina, make you calmer, and generally improve your health at all levels.

9

Beat Fatigue with Meditation

If you meditate every day you are going to have more energy, vigour and stamina. But there are other reasons why you should meditate – these are just the 'side-effects' of meditation, an additional bonus. In Chapter 2, I explained that there are eight limbs of yoga: different elements that include the yoga postures and yoga breathing. Meditation, the seventh limb, is about finding your real self and your real truth. If you are not interested in doing this, that's fine, but you will benefit in lots of other ways because meditation can:

- calm the mind
- help you to feel relaxed
- relieve anxiety and help to take away worries
- relieve insomnia
- slow down the production of stress-related chemicals and your breathing and heart-rate
- give stamina and raise energies
- heal
- reduce information overload in the brain and give you some space
- help to bring your mind under control so that your thoughts and emotions do not sweep you along
- help you to feel more centred and balanced
- bring peace and a sense of purpose to your life

- help you to find your own truth and to get in touch with your real self

This is quite a long list of benefits, and even if you are interested in only some of them, you can perhaps see why meditation is so popular today. However, unless you are very lucky, meditation is not usually something that just happens, or that you just 'do'. It's not as easy as just clearing your mind and not thinking for 20 minutes. In fact if you try to do this you will probably find it impossible – your mind will start buzzing with thoughts and ideas. Meditation requires practice and discipline. Later in this chapter I shall give you some guidelines so that you can learn how to start meditating. In the meantime I'm going to explain a bit more about the mind and why meditation can help *you*.

Meditation is said to take place when everything stops. It is the stopping – stilling your mind and listening in to silence – that is difficult. Meditation is about being able to let go of your thoughts – not by forcing them out or trying to drive them away, but by allowing them to come and go without getting involved in them. Let's think about this for a moment. It is the nature of the mind always to be active, flitting from one thing to another. This is incredibly exhausting because you are dissipating prana or vital energy as you move from one thought to another in a split second in your busy and noisy mind. Your mind *loves* being active; it is rather like a runaway chariot, with your thoughts being the out of control horses running in all directions, and you the charioteer trying to rein them in. In this way, you may find that you are swept along in life by your feeling and emotions. As I said in Chapter 2, yoga and meditation is about *control* of the thought waves of your mind. Think about how one thought triggers another, then another and another, like a chain. In yoga it is believed that this thought-chain, or unruly mind, is the root of all trouble and disease – and, of course, exhaustion. The first step in meditation is to be *aware* of your busy mind, of this chain, so that you can learn to let it go and not become involved in it. In this way meditation will help you to bring all your scattered energy back to one point.

Meditation is also about exploring your *real* self so that you can learn to put aside your everyday thoughts and desires. It's a bit like peeling back layers of an onion skin to find out who you really are. As you start meditating you may well find that it feels rather like coming home, as if you are coming back to something you are very familiar with. If you continue to meditate regularly you will feel a sense of deep calm, relaxation and peace. This is because in your everyday activities and thinking your brainwaves occur in spiky, fast Theta waves. When you meditate, these brainwaves change to the slower Alpha waves associated with relaxation. Eventually you may experience even slower Delta waves, similar to those in sleep, which indicate a very deep level of relaxation. This of course is very restful, and as a consequence your energy will be boosted at the end of your session.

HOW TO MEDITATE

You may be surprised to realize that there already is an element of meditation in your life. For example, if you are really concentrating on reading a book, driving your car or doing anything that involves your mind in a disciplined way so that it doesn't wander off into the 'chain' of thinking I mentioned earlier, you are laying the foundation for learning to meditate. If you are doing an activity such as yoga postures, gardening, painting, listening to music, walking in the countryside or watching a beautiful sunset, try and rein in your mind so that it is engrossed in just this one activity. To get the idea of this, really focus on your everyday tasks and try not to flit from one thing to another. Think only about what you are doing and really absorb yourself in the present moment without fantasizing or worrying about anything else. In this way you are learning to concentrate and not wasting energy on superfluous thinking.

Preparation

To start meditating, you need to do the following:

- Find a quiet place where you will not be interrupted. The room should be warm and you should meditate in the same place at the same time every day so that you create a routine.
- Do not meditate for at least two hours after a meal, or if you are sleepy.
- The best time to meditate is first thing in the morning, at noon, or at sunset.
- If possible, sit with your spine upright, because you are working with vertical energies. If for any reason you cannot do this, lie down.
- Sit comfortably, either on a chair with your feet on the floor, or on the floor cross-legged or in the half-lotus position.
- Hold your hands palms upwards with your forefinger and thumb touching – or place them on your knees.
- Do not try to meditate after frenzied activity – you won't succeed! Try doing some yoga postures or yoga breathing first.
- Aim to put all your cares and worries aside for the duration of your meditation. This is *your* time and you don't need to think about anything else. Use the pigeonhole visualization explained in Chapter 5 if you find this helpful.
- Breathe rhythmically and slowly from your diaphragm.
- You may like to imagine a white light surrounding and protecting you during your session.
- Try to close off your senses. Ignore any outside stimulation, any outside sounds you may hear. Try and turn your attention inwards. Look, with your eyes closed, at the point between your eyebrows.
- Focus on a single point, such as the rhythm of your breath.
- Meditate for 10 minutes a day at first, then gradually increase this time to 20 minutes.
- When you have finished you need to ground yourself. Never come out of meditation suddenly. Stay where you are. Wriggle

your spine into your chair or onto the floor. Shake your hands. Slowly stretch your limbs.

- Finally, meditation needs both intention and effort; it isn't something that just happens. It may take you weeks, months or even longer to see the benefits, so practise, practise, practise. The results will be well worth the effort.

DIFFERENT WAYS TO MEDITATE

Creative Meditation

Creative meditation is an excellent way to start. It involves thinking about one word, which you can then build on within the boundaries of that concept. For example, you take an idea or theme such as Love, Peace, Harmony, Health, God or Energy, which you then hold in your mind. You continue by thinking only about words relating to that theme during your practice. You should use only constructive or positive words so that your energies are led upwards – destructive or selfish thinking will lead to fear, anxiety and exhaustion.

Exercise
Select one of the above words that I suggested. Now sit quietly for ten minutes with your eyes closed and concentrate on this word or things associated with this word. In this way you can build up ideas from your chosen word. For example, if you chose the word Love you may think of joy, happiness, your family, and so on. The difficult thing is to keep focused on your chosen theme, building up ideas on the word but not letting your mind wander on to other ideas away from your chosen theme. This isn't easy, I know, but don't give up! If your mind starts to wander, bring it back gently to ideas about the word you have chosen. Don't try to force your mind; if unrelated thoughts enter your mind just observe them and let them go without becoming involved in their chain. Don't get frustrated if you find this difficult.

Now review what happened. Did you feel uncomfortable? Did outside sounds disturb you? Did your mind wander off? If it did, don't be disheartened; keep practising and eventually you will find that your mind starts to become stiller, which in turn will give you a deep sense of calm and more energy.

Concentration

Concentration is said to be the brickwork of meditation. It is about keeping your mind focused on only one thing, so that it is one-pointed and not dissipated. If you can focus on just one seed, such as a word or image, you can start to still your mind and turn your attention inwards, which leads on to meditation. I mentioned earlier that it will help if you live your life by focusing on the present moment and not jumping from one pursuit to another. This in turn will help your concentration. Using the analogy of a wheel, I can explain by saying that if you live your life on the rim you will rush about from one experience to the next, trying to find happiness and contentment. However, if you return to the still, peaceful centre of the wheel, you will find that this contentment comes from *inside* yourself, rather than from the pursuit of external objects. By turning your concentration and your attention inwards, you focus your mind on your inner world, where you will find a state of peace – whatever happens to you. Concentration and meditation will take you away from activities which involve disturbance, confusion and restlessness. This is why meditation can give you energy.

Concentration is not as easy as it sounds, but when learning to meditate it usually takes the form of following the breath, or concentrating on an image or word. Or you can use a mantra, a sound with meaning.

Exercises

You may like to try all the suggestions given here for learning to concentrate, but once you have found one that suits you I suggest you stick to it and use the same method every day.

1 Using your *breath* is a powerful way to achieve concentration. Sit quietly with your eyes closed for ten minutes. Start by focusing on the natural rhythm of your breathing. Observe it but don't force it, just let it happen naturally. You can try any of the following:

- Concentrating on your breathing, count mentally from one to four on each in-breath. If your mind wanders and you forget to count, bring your attention back to the natural rhythm of your breath and start at one again.
- Just watch your breath, focusing on the feeling as it comes in and out of your nostrils. Feel how it is cool as you breathe in and warmer as you exhale. Notice any sibilant sound it makes. Watch the rise and fall of your diaphragm. Focus on the space between your breaths. Notice the stillness. Hear the silence.
- You can use the traditional Ham Sa breathing mantra. Mentally say 'Ham' as you breath in and 'Sa' as you breath out. Ham Sa is called the natural mantra because it's repeated by every living thing that breathes.

2 A *mantra* (a single word or short phrase) is another powerful tool for concentration. The sound and vibration of a mantra channel energy and help the mind to become focused. Traditional mantras are carefully constructed to purify and transform.

Aum, or Om, which is said to be the sound of the whole of the universe, is one of the best mantras to start with. It is beneficial at a very profound level if practised every day and can bring about changes in your life quite rapidly, because it helps you to tune into your real self. Om is also very balancing; it massages the vital organs, increases blood flow, stimulates the nervous system and relaxes the respiratory system (*see* Chapter 3).

Another traditional mantra you may like to try is 'Om mani padme hum'. This means the 'Jewel in the Heart of the Lotus', but the vibration and rhythm of the words are just as effective as their meaning.

You can chose your own mantra, but whatever word or phrase you use, immerse yourself in the sound and become absorbed in it. You can say it out loud or silently, in time with your breath.

3 You can concentrate on an *object* such as a candle flame, a flower or a roaring fire. Or you may like to pick an image that has significance for you, such as the Cross, the Buddha or the Om symbol (*see* figure 42). Having studied your chosen object, close your eyes and focus on it with your mind's eye for ten minutes. If your attention wanders, open you eyes, look at the object, then close them again.

4 *Yoga postures* can be a form of meditation in themselves. When you hold a yoga posture and focus only on that, your mind is kept within the boundaries of the task in hand and will start to become still. This is why yoga is often called *action in inaction*. So if you want to prepare for meditation, you can make a start by concentrating on each yoga position as you hold it, without allowing your mind to wander.

Figure 42   The Symbol for Om

Receptive Meditation

If you have practised the above exercises for some time you may now like to try stilling your mind. By this I don't mean that you should empty your mind but, rather, that you observe your thoughts without getting involved in them, and without following the 'thought chain'. If you try to push your thoughts away too hard you will give them energy, so please don't worry if you find this difficult. It takes time and perseverance to still your mind. When you meditate you lose thoughts of 'I' or 'mine' – and this is something you can't force. It may take weeks or months, or it may just happen!

EXERCISES

1 Sit quietly for 10–20 minutes with your eyes closed, as described earlier under Preparation. Think of your mind as a calm pool, with no ripples. If thoughts occur, observe them and let them go, but don't become involved. If your attention wanders, bring it back by listening to the silence between your breaths.
2 Visualize a stormy sea gradually calming down until it becomes smooth and quiet. The sea is your mind, and as it becomes quiet, listen to the vibrant presence of the silence. Keep your awareness in the present moment so that your thoughts are neither supressed nor encouraged, just witnessed.

I said at the beginning of this chapter that meditation is about controlling the thought waves of the mind, and I also explained how this could then release great energy. Meditation is really about replacing the thoughts that arise from desires, restlessness and dissatisfaction with thoughts of harmony and contentment. In this way you will find not only more energy but also inner peace. Meditation will lead you back to your true nature and help you to still your mind so that you are in control.

10

My Story

I'd like to finish this book by telling you something about myself – and my own personal knowledge of fatigue and how this brought me to yoga. Everything I've written about in this book is taken from my own experience, which is why I *know* that yoga can beat fatigue.

I suffered from the most severe form of fatigue (myalgic encephalomyelitis (ME) – sometimes known as Chronic Fatigue Syndrome or CFS) before yoga helped me in my recovery. In 1989 I was running a successful public relations company. My job was very stressful and I worked very long hours. I didn't take lunch breaks or holidays and I often worked at weekends. In order to prop up my flagging energy levels I ate lots of junk food, including sweets and chocolate. When I went home I would drink a bottle of wine to numb the exhaustion and slow down my racing brain, and I would heat up a ready-prepared meal in the microwave.

The first warning I got that all was not well was panic attacks. For no apparent reason I would start to feel shaky, anxious and very strange – as if I wasn't really there – and I would have difficulty getting my breath. This was followed by chronic insomnia; sometimes I went for two or three nights without sleep. I thought the answer was to ignore the distress signals my body was sending me and to work harder. I also joined an aerobics class, which I squeezed into my lunch hour. The fatigue was incredible – I was *always* tired – but I just ignored the exhaustion and got on with running my business. In fact, I didn't really think about the fatigue – I just assumed that it was normal, that life was like that and it was something I just had to accept. Then I got what I thought was flu. After three days in bed, I dragged myself back to work. I was exhausted and dizzy, but I thought I had to work or my world would cave in. My doctor took some blood tests and later told me I had glandular fever, also known as the Epstein—Barr virus. She advised me to rest, so I slowed down a bit – but not enough. Six months later I sold my business. I started work as a television researcher but then noticed some more unnerving symptoms that I couldn't ignore. The exhaustion would get so bad that sometimes I couldn't even speak, and I would have to go and lie down. On one occasion my husband found me on the floor in the dining room – I couldn't move! If I rested, I was still tired; even when I woke up I was tired. I managed to struggle on with my job, even if it meant lying down in the lunch hour rather than socializing with the others in the production team. I existed on chocolate for a quick boost of energy, but that soon wore off. Eventually I became so ill that I had to give up work. Resting didn't make me any better and if I exercised it took me days to recover. My muscles ached, I had a permanent fog in my head, and the insomnia got worse. Eventually, in 1990, I was diagnosed as suffering from ME/CFS. If only I had listened to my body when it had first sent me signals to slow down!

My health deteriorated until, in 1992, I was in a wheelchair. At this point I was too tired even to hold a conversation. Simple things like making a cup of tea were like climbing a mountain, and if I over-exerted myself it would take days to recover. I was taken into hospital for three months and put on various drugs. Still I made little progress. I did, however, meet a wonderful woman called Nancy Farley who introduced me to meditation. In 1993 my local yoga teacher, Angela Stevens, asked me if I would help her set up a yoga group for people with ME. She had noticed that this was a common problem and thought remedial yoga would help. I wasn't so sure – strenuous exercise was the last thing I needed – but Angela assured me yoga wasn't like that. So I got together a group of people and we started. Almost immediately I began to feel better. Angela concentrated on yoga breathing, relaxation and meditation. There were some gentle stretching exercises to get our systems going and to start to build up the muscle groups, but we took these very slowly and at our own pace. Sometimes I over estimated my health and did too much, but that was usually because I was trying to keep up with someone on a higher level of ability. The first rule of yoga is 'work within your own limits'!

I started visiting the UK Yoga for Health Foundation – the largest yoga residential centre in Europe. They were doing a lot of work with ME and CFS as well as with general tiredness and stress – and I learned more about the importance of proper diet and meditation. Since yoga has become part of my life I have much more energy, I think positively all the time, and I look at what I have rather than what I don't have. When I am well, I really appreciate my health and give thanks for it – and I focus on what I am able to do rather than get angry about what I can't do. I accept that this is how things are for now. Most of the time, however, I have more energy than I did before I was ill – providing I pace my activities. Best of all, I feel I have spiritual direction, something which my previous lifestyle had made me ignore. I am still recovering and have to be careful not to overdo things, but am now able to participate in an intermediate yoga class. I think this is wonderful considering I was in a wheelchair a few years ago.

Whenever I visit the Yoga for Health Foundation, I am always amazed at the stories of other people – many of whom were also very disabled by ME/CFS but have now recovered completely, thanks to adopting a yoga lifestyle. Although mine is an extreme story, this book was written not just for people with CFS, but for *everyone* who suffers from fatigue or exhaustion. So if you are suffering from a lack of energy, or tired all the time, just think how quickly you could see results by practising yoga and making it part of your everyday routine!

SUMMARY

Here's a reminder of the main points of this book – the things you might like to try to Beat Fatigue with Yoga!

- Firstly, be aware of your health. Start to tune in to how you feel every day.
- Practise some yoga postures regularly – especially the Pose of Complete Rest.
- Take enough rest and relaxation and make time for yourself.
- Check your posture regularly.
- Eat as nutritious a diet as you can.
- Drink lots of water.
- Practise breathing slowly and rhythmically using your diaphragm.
- Try using some of the special yoga breathing exercises from Chapter 4.
- Sit outside in the fresh air and sunshine, visit the seaside or the mountains, and walk barefoot to take in extra prana whenever possible.
- Avoid pollution, dust and smoke as these zap vital energy.
- Meditate for 10–20 minutes every day.
- Take responsibility for your own health – some of us treat our cars better than our bodies! Respect yourself and your health.
- Remember, positive thinking raises prana, so try and see the good things in your life and don't focus on the bad things.

Good Luck!

Glossary

Prana	Universal Life Energy
Asana	Yoga posture
Pranayama	Yoga breathing
Chakra	Energy centre in the body
Nadi	Channel for vital energy
Mantra	A word, phrase or sound which has meaning
Bandha	A position used to lock in energy
Mudra	A hand position to direct energy flow

Bibliography

Ajaya, Swami, *Yoga Psychology*, The Himalayan International Institute of Yoga Science and Philosophy, 1976

Bell, Lorna, and Seyfer, Eudora, *Gentle Yoga*, Celestial Arts, 1982

Brennan, Barbara, *Light Emerging*, Bantam, 1993

Brennan, Barbara, *Hands of Light*, Bantam, 1987

Carter, Jill, and Edwards, Alison, *The Elimination Diet Cookbook*, Element Books, 1997

Carter, Jill, and Edwards, Alison, *The Rotation Diet Cookbook*, Element Books, 1997

Capra, Fritjof, *The Tao of Physics*, Flamingo, 1982

Chaitow, Leon, *The Beat Fatigue Workbook*, Thorsons, 1988

Crawford, Moira, *The Natural Way with Allergies*, Element Books, 1997

Devereux, Godfrey, *The Elements of Yoga*, Element Books, 1994

Eastcott, Michal, *The Silent Path*, Rider, 1989

Freedman, Miriam, and Hankes, Janice, *Yoga at Work*, Element Books, 1996

Heilbronn, Bill, *The Yoga Students' Companion*, published by the author, 1995

Isaacson, Cheryl, *Thorsons Principles of Yoga*, Thorsons, 1996

Iyengar, B S K, *Light on Yoga*, Thorsons, 1991

Jacobs, Gill, *The Natural Way: Chronic Fatigue Syndrome*, Element Books 1997

Jacobs, Gill, and Joanna Kjaer *Beat Candida Through Diet*, Vermillion, 1997

Kelder, Peter, *Tibetan Secrets of Youth and Vitality*, Thorsons, 1988

Kent, Howard, *Breathe Better, Feel Better*, Apple Press, 1997

Kent, Howard, *The Complete Yoga Course*, Headline, 1995

Martin, Simon *The Natural Way with Candida*, Element Books, 1998

Mehta, Silva, Mira and Shyam, *Yoga the Iyengar Way*, Dorling Kindersely, 1995

Muktananda, Swami, *Where are you Going?*, Gurudev Siddha
     Peeth, 1982
Nagarathna, Dr R, Nagendra, Dr H R, and Monro, Dr R, *Yoga for
     Common Ailments*, Gaia Books, 1990
Ozaniec, Naomi, *The Elements of the Chakras*, Element Books, 1996
Page, Dr Christine, *Frontiers of Health*, The C W Daniel Company
     Ltd, 1996
Purna, Dr Svami, *Yoga, a Practical Introduction*, Element Books, 1998
Ramacharaka, Yogi, *The Hindu Yogi Science of Breath*, L N Fowler and Co
     Ltd, 1960
Sears, Barry, *Enter the Zone*, Regan Books, 1995
Sivananda, Swami, *The Science of Pranayama*, The Divine Life
     Society, 1992
Sivananda Yoga Centre, *The Book of Yoga*, Ebury Press, 1995
Smith, Erica, and Wilks, Nicholas, *Meditation*, Vermillion, 1997
Stewart, Dr Alan, *Tired All the Time*, Optima, 1993
Sturgess, Stephen, *The Yoga Book*, Element Books, 1997
Tobias, Maxine, and Stewart, Mary, *Stretch and Relax*, Dorling
     Kindersley, 1995
Van Lysebeth, Andre, *Pranayama*, Unwin, 1983
Vollmar V, *Journey Through the Chakras*, Gateway Books, 1992
White, Ruth, *Working with Your Chakras*, Piatkus, 1993
Yogananda, Sri Sri Paramhansa, *Autobiography of a Yogi*, Jaico
     Publishing House, 1975

Useful Addresses

THE YOGA FOR HEALTH FOUNDATION

The Yoga For Health Foundation trains teachers and has yoga clubs in the following countries:

Australia
PO Box 313
Montville
Queensland 4560

Barbados
PO Box 21A
Brittons Hill
St Michael's

Belgium
Ridder van Ranstlei 16
B 2050 Mortsel

Canada
2121 Galena Crescent
Oakville
Ontario L6H 4A9

1562 Southdown Road
Mississanga
Ontario L5J 2Z4

Denmark
Bgevonget 112
8310 Tranbjerg

Egypt
15 Abdel Khaler Sarwat
St Laurens
Alexandria

Eire
117 Gaybrook Lawns
Malahide
Co Dublin

Germany
Kienbachstr 22
82211 Herrsching

Holland
Reestraat 3
1016 DM
Amsterdam

Hong Kong
6B Victoria Court
Ville de Cascade
2-4 Lai Wo Lane
Fotan, Shatin

Israel
Smuts 17
62009 Tel Aviv

Lithuania
Paberzes 14-100
Vilnius 2010

New Zealand
37 Te Henga Road
Henderson RD1
Auckland

Poland
Nawojowa 33-335
Woj Nowy Sacz

Portugal
370 Vale Do Lobo
Almancil
Algarve

Romania
Str. Progresului 8
Sc. 3 Ap. 23
Onesti 5450

Russia
Bld 40/12, app 55
Novatorov's Street
117421
Moscow

South Africa
4 Barry Road
Pietermaritzburg 3021

Spain
Aparto Num 5
Cazorla, Jaen

UK
Ickwell Bury
Nr Biggleswade
Bedfordshire SG18 9EF
England

The UK Foundation also runs various residential courses, including those for fatigue, and has books and tapes for sale. Write for details of courses or about becoming a member.

USA
7918 Bolling Drive
Alexandria VA 22308

CFS / ME

If you have Chronic Fatigue Syndrome or ME and would like help and support, the following organizations offer fact sheets, advice lines and a membership journal.

Australia
Anzymes
Po Box 7
Moonee Ponds
Victoria 3039

ME Association
Stanhope House
High Street
Stanford-le-Hope
Essex SS17 0HA

New Zealand
Anzymes (NZ) Inc
PO Box 35–429
Browns Bay
Auckland 10

USA
The CFIDS Association of America
Inc
PO Box 220398
Charlotte NC 28222-0398

South Africa
ME Association of South Africa
PO Box 461
Hillcrest 3650
Natal

National CFS Association
3521 Broadway-Suite 222
Kansas City,
Missouri 64111

UK
Action for ME
PO Box 1302
Wells
Somerset BA5 1YE

OTHER RESOURCES

Specialist in nutritional and environmental medicine:

Dr Jonathan Briffa
The Executive Suite
Cannons, Cousins Lane
London EC4A
Tel: 0171 283 0105

The British Wheel of Yoga

1 Hamilton Place
Boston Road
Wells
Somerset BA5 1YE

Tapes/Yoga Classes for CFS sufferers:

Angela Stevens
Laminga
Southview Road
Wadhurst
E. Sussex TN5 6TL
England

Two tapes available – *Yoga, the Gentle Way* and *Breathe to Live*. For details and an up-to-date list of teachers who specialize in yoga for CFS, send a s.a.e. to the above address.

Index